The Psychology Behind Fitness Motivation:

A Revolutionary New Program to Lose Weight and Stay Fit for Life

I0426583

First published 2013
By Dr. Kim Chronister
The Psychology Behind Fitness Motivation:
A Revolutionary New Program to Lose Weight and Stay Fit for Life
©2013 Dr. Kim Chronister

ISBN-10: 1493709836
ISBN-13: 978-1493709830
Printed at Createspace.com
(United States of America)

Legal Disclaimer

This book's information is meant to supplement, not replace, physical activity training in its proper form. All forms of exercise pose some inherent risks.

The publisher as well as the editors advise readers to take full and proper responsibility for their safety and acknowledge their limits. Prior to practicing the physical activity exercises in this book, ensure that your equipment is suitable and well-maintained. Be advised to refrain from taking any risks beyond your level of fitness experience, training, and aptitude. The dietary and physical activity programs in this book are not intended as a substitute for any physical activity routine or dietary regimen that might have been prescribed by your doctor. As with all physical activity exercises and dietary programs, it is highly recommended that you first seek your doctor's approval before beginning a new regimen.

Contents

Part III   Adopting the Fitness Motivation Mentality

Part IV   Extras

Acknowledgments

When it comes to thanking people, I always think of my mom first. My mom has always been my real-life hero. Her love and devotion to her children remain an inspiration. I miss my mom every day. Thank you to my dad, who was so happy to have me, and who taught me so many valuable lessons. I am so grateful for my entire family, especially my brothers Matt and Chris, my special grandparents, and my two wonderful aunties. Thank you also to all of my close friends that are family as well to me. Special thanks to Griselda Noriega for your endless support. Thank you to Dr. Ramani Durvasula (author of *You Are Why You Eat*) and Dr. Joan Murray (my inspirational professor) for your endless help with my dissertation from which this book was inspired. Finally, thank you to every individual who has ever reached out to me. You have made me a better person and better at helping others.

"The Psychology Behind Fitness Motivation helps you move past your previous limitations and embrace the body and vitality you've always wanted."

- Dr. John Spencer Ellis

Dr. John Spencer Ellis is the founder of NESTA (National Exercise and Sports Trainers Association (NESTA) and Wexford University.

Introduction:

FITNESS MOTIVATION TO GET FIT AND STAY FIT FOR LIFE

This is a book for the unmotivated, for those who have been fit and long to be fit again, and for those of you who have never been fit with the desire to attain the body and health of your dreams. This book is also for those of you who need motivation that will last longer than you ever imagined and a realistic path toward fitness and fitness motivation based on evidence-based research that works. I am a health psychologist and a wellness expert with years of experience transforming minds and bodies. I have dedicated my life's research to helping those in need of fitness motivation, weight loss, and an overall healthy self-image.

How I Developed the Program

While working on my doctoral degree in clinical psychology, I became a certified personal trainer and helped many clients transform their minds and bodies for the better. During our training sessions, I discovered that although the cardio and strength training was essential for their weight loss goals, *a lot of their success depended on our discussions about the way they felt about themselves, their self-talk, and their dedication to the process.*

I am certain that you are aware of the high cost of hiring a personal trainer (especially one that comes to your home). I realize that not all of you live in Beverly Hills and can afford the luxuries of a personal trainer for life; and even if you are from a wealthy area and have plenty of monetary resources, I truly believe that one misses out on a major benefit of the attainment of fitness if one does not become self-motivated. If you do intend on hiring a personal trainer, I will let you in on what to tell them in the beginning so that by the end of your time together, you will be left empowered rather than disempowered. I feel strongly that there is something much more fulfilling about acquiring autonomy and self-empowerment when it comes to being fit. Research shows that autonomy plays a significant role in a person's ability to be motivated and stay motivated to engage in physical activity in the long-term.

When my research of the psychology of fitness was completed for the dissertation, I discovered that empowerment was a giant factor in long-term outcomes with regard to keeping weight off and continuing on a fitness regimen. For this reason, I began recommending shorter (2 to 3 month) personal training programs so that the client could learn the workouts and feel empowered to do them on their own for life.

I remember (during personal training sessions) secretly wishing that I could teach my clients everything I know about motivation to become physically fit and how to work out to attain, and maintain, their desired weight loss goals. However, many clients had not *yet* aligned their self-talk with that of someone who works out on their own several times a week. During a workout, a client would say, "You know I wouldn't do this on my own," or "I couldn't have gotten through this workout without you," or "I would never do this many sit ups if you weren't watching me." If you can relate to any of the previously noted statements, you will soon learn how to utilize cognitive behavioral techniques to reframe these types of thoughts that are preventing you from the ability to motivate yourself for the rest of your life.

The relationships that I built with my clients and the discussions we shared led me to examine the ways in which thoughts, and how we handle emotions, affect behavior; and more specifically, how our thoughts affect whether or not we are able to become self-motivated to achieve and maintain our fitness goals. For this reason, I consulted experts in the field of psychology who are well-versed in cognitive behavioral interventions.

Dr. Ramani Durvasula (author of *You are Why You Eat*) and Dr. Joan Murray (associate professor at Alliant International University) kindly accepted my invitation to consult with me on my dissertation. Dr. Durvasula and Dr. Murray made invaluable contributions to the project and helped me uncover how to motivate depressed clients to engage in physical activity. *While writing the dissertation, I realized that a great deal of this research is applicable to people with and without mood disorders who simply desire the motivation to engage in regular physical activity.* As a result, I decided to write my dissertation about the psychology of fitness motivation that was later turned into the book that you are now reading.

What This Program Was Designed to Do For You

Despite the known benefits of physical activity, only 25 percent of Americans participate in physical activity at the recommended level (by the CDC, the AHA, the ACSM, and the US Surgeon General) according to behavioral risk factor surveys. As a result, a large proportion of American adults don't participate in regular fitness routines and, thus, do not benefit from the positive mental health effects of exercise. *This program will teach you clinically and scientifically proven motivational techniques. These techniques will motivate you and help you*:

▶ Handle negative emotions and stress-related symptoms effectively

▶ Improve your overall health

▶ Control your mind and body and heighten peace of mind

▶ Think more positively and optimistically, which is a trait recognized as improving physical health

▶ Realize the powerful effect your mind has on your emotions and health and that you have the ability to realize the strength that is within you

▶ Feel confident and ready to embrace new opportunities

▶ Visualize yourself as an athlete

▶ Attain your weight loss goals/fitness goals

▶ And much more

I strongly believe in balance when it comes to workouts. I also believe in mixing up your workouts, staying excited about your fitness goals, and learning what works for you so that you avoid burn out and stick to your goals for life. There is nothing empowering about feeling defeated at the end of a workout. For this reason, realistic weight loss and muscle-building goals must be set. I offer a balanced fitness plan in this book. This plan has been created for the purpose of being able to stay with a fitness regimen for life.

In addition to the fitness plan that is provided for you in this book, the tools that will help you on your way toward fitness motivation come from evidence-based interventions, including such interventions as cognitive behavioral therapy (CBT) and motivational interviewing (MI). Both CBT and MI interventions are proven to motivate clients and lead them toward success in their fitness goals.

In my work as a therapist, I have utilized cognitive behavioral therapy and motivational interviewing to increase adaptive exercise behaviors. I chose to write this book not only because of its relevance to my clinical work but also because of my *sincere* interest in physical activity promotion for those of you in need of fitness motivation for mood enhancement, attainment of weight loss goals, and overall life enhancement.

At the core, the number one tip for making this program effective for you (for weight loss and staying motivated for fitness for life) is asserting a commitment to yourself to become happy; and because you are making a commitment to be happy, you will likely attract plenty of positive things to your life. For the first time ever, or for the first time in a long while, you will feel great about yourself. There's a lot of work to do, every day is a process, and you must contribute by putting the program into practice. Though this may not be the easiest program, the outcome-increased mind-body control, greater control over your emotions, a more positive outlook, better health and well-being, and the body you deserve-*make this program one of the best investments in your life.*

This book is not just about obtaining fitness motivation. By learning to work out regularly, you will also feel more energy and joy, feel more confident, more optimistic, and cope better with life's stressors. You will enjoy being around others and they will enjoy being around you. There are endless possibilities of life improvements that can occur after learning and applying the valuable and evidenced-based tools for you in this program. *This program is designed for you to obtain the body, health, and happiness you have always desired.*

PART I
Getting Started

Chapter One

SAY GOODBYE TO YOUR "BEFORE" BODY

Your "before" body is a product of past thoughts and behaviors. From this point on, you will be able to see yourself as a fitness junkie, an athlete, a person who feels less like yourself without your regular work out. Exercise will become your go-to stress relief, cathartic alone time or even your time to socialize if you choose to work out in the company of others. You can think of working out similarly to showering. Your day begins and sometimes ends with it, you feel more confident because you did it, and you are giving yourself the proper preparation for a great day. You wouldn't go a day without showering (and if you did, you wouldn't feel at your best). You will learn to regulate your mood and emotions with exercise. Stress will be much easier to handle and dealing with emotions caused by life hurdles such as work and interpersonal issues will be much more tolerable.

Many people do not engage in enough physical activity and, as a result, are not able to benefit from the mood-elevating effects caused by regular exercise. Depressed individuals often struggle to maintain the motivation necessary to participate in regular physical activity. Although working out may be beneficial to their mental health, it is difficult for most people who are feeling down to find the motivation necessary to comply with a physical activity regimen. A significant lack of physical activity in a person's routine has been correlated with enhanced risk for depression. In addition to using negative self-talk, depressed individuals often lack the motivation necessary to change their behaviors. Depression makes it difficult for people to begin, or adhere to, recommendations given to them by mental health professionals. In addition, depression can contribute to an individual's lack of motivation due to such issues as significantly depressed mood, lack of interest in most of their previous and typical activities, and low energy. *Thus (as previously discussed), depressed clients are way less likely to participate in healthy behaviors, such as physical activity.*

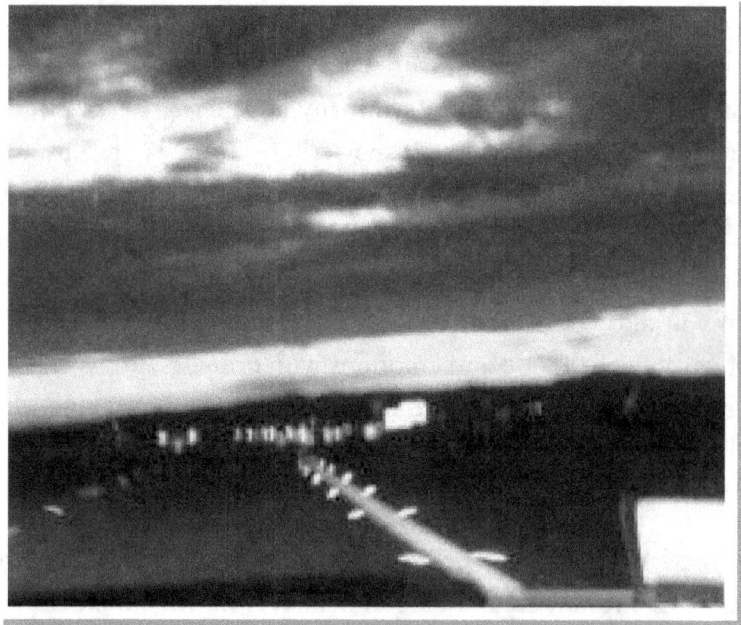

Making changes to one's behavior (such as working out) can be an effective natural depression treatment. Moreover, most research show that the mood improvement effect of physical activity can most likely be similar to that of traditional psychotherapy and psychiatric medication. Whether you relate to feelings of depression or not, your negative emotions may be reflected in your "before" body.

Stages of Change

The famous and easy to understand stages of change model (created by Prochaska and DiClemente's) can provide theoretical support for this wellness program to promote physical activity. According to this behavioral change model, behavior change happens as individuals move through stages of readiness for change. The stages in this model that are helpful in establishing where you are in change are pre-contemplation (earliest), contemplation (considering change soon), preparation (self-explanatory), action (the exciting stage), and maintenance (long-term).

Pre-contemplation is the earliest stage of behavior change. In this stage, people are not even thinking about changing in the next six months and they have no intention to change as of yet. If you fall into the pre-contemplation stage, you may not even be aware that your lack of regular activity is unhealthy or you may feel defeated from past failed attempts.

Contemplation is the behavior change stage where people are contemplating changing within the next six months. In this stage, people are acknowledging that there is a problem. However, they are not yet ready or certain of wanting to make a change. If you fall into this middle stage, you may be just starting to think about increasing your physical activity behaviors.

Preparation is the behavior change stage where people are planning to take action in the near future, typically within one month. If you fall within this stage, you are getting ready to increase your levels of physical activity. If and/or when you fall into this stage, I would like to congratulate you on your decision to make one of the most essential changes of behavior in your life.

Action is a stage where people make specific changes with regards to behavior. This stage is all about willpower. It is about changing behavior (in this case working out regularly and consistently). If you fall into the action stage, you have begun to take action to increase your healthy behaviors.

Finally, **maintenance** is the stage of change in which clients are working on relapse prevention (in this case working on maintaining engagement in regular physical activity and preventing a relapse into not working out regularly). If you are in this final stage, you have made a change, you are working out regularly, and you are working hard to keep it up.

A willingness to change and readiness are major factors in a client's success in a wellness program such as this one. It is beneficial for those of you who need help to become motivated to exercise regularly to determine your readiness change as well as integrate the stages of change throughout the process. *Each individual must decide for him or herself when a stage is completed and the appropriate time to move on to the next stage.* The decision to move onto the next stage must come from inside you in order for you to feel a sense of control and autonomy making you more likely to continue conquering your goals.

Why This Program Is Different

The physiological health benefits of physical fitness activity have been researched by scientists and researchers extensively. Despite this fact, less research has been dedicated to the psychological benefits of physical activity and the most effective ways to promote physical activity. This program is based on inter-ventions that have been clinically proven to help individuals become motivated to engage in regular physical activity. These interventions include cognitive behavioral therapy, motivation-al interviewing, and additional interventions recommended targeting those in need of fitness motivation. When equipped with the proper tools, anyone can become self-motivated to engage in regular exercise. The purpose of this program is to educate those in need of fitness motivation about the benefits of exercise and ways to become self-motivated.

This program achieves its remarkable results because it is based on evidenced-based interventions. In most cases, the causes of a lack of fitness motivation are thoughts and behaviors that are learned and can be unlearned. Some examples include:

▶ Negative beliefs about ability to engage in physical activity

▶ Feeling out of control of one's own life

▶ Negative responses to feelings of stress and sadness

▶ Overall neglect of physical health

▶ Negative thinking about oneself

Interventions Used in This Program that Will Make You Motivated

The following information addresses the most effective ways that mental health professionals promote physical activity in depressed clients. These techniques can be used for anyone struggling with a lack of motivation to exercise. The specific ways in which health psychologists, like myself, and other mental health professionals help to promote exercise among these clients include Cognitive Behavioral Therapy (CBT) and Motivational Interviewing (M.I.). Both M.I. and CBT are evidence-based treatments which translate into appropriate interventions for motivating individuals to engage in physical activity. CBT is a proven treatment for behavioral change and M.I. can be used to improve motivation to change among those seeking motivation to exercise on a regular basis. Both M.I. and CBT can be effective in facilitating long-term behavioral change as it pertains to exercise.

Cognitive Behavioral Therapy (CBT) is a commonly used and remarkable treatment for depressive disorder, anxiety disorders, and other psychological issues. CBT encompasses a use of cognitive therapy (a focus on identifying and altering dysfunctional cognitions and beliefs) and behavior therapy (a focus on using techniques obtained from behavioral principles of classical and operant conditioning). A cognitive-behavioral approach for promoting behavior change such as exercising more frequently is goal-oriented, present-centered, and time-limited.

Since CBT is goal-oriented, it will be simple to focus on positive outcomes of your new weight loss promoting behaviors and look forward to new events. CBT is also present-centered so it makes no difference of how little your motivation was previously or that you hadn't been working out as much as you would like before reading this book. It only matters how you choose to identify now (as a fitness junkie, an athlete, and/or someone who craves their daily work out). Since CBT is time-limited, you will be able to learn new techniques to become, and stay, motivated and be on your way to becoming self-motivated in a short amount of time.

One important evidence-based intervention currently receiving a significant amount of interest is **Motivational**

Interviewing (M.I.). M.I. has been shown to be highly effective when it's combined with other proven and remarkable treatment methods such as cognitive behavioral therapy. *For this reason, I have combined both CBT and M.I. in this program for the purpose of providing the most effective method for those of you in need of fitness motivation.*

Motivational interviewing is a client-centered technique used to improve intrinsic motivation for change by processing and eliminating ambivalence. Ambivalence is the conflict individuals experience when exploring the costs and benefits of engaging in a particular behavior. An example of ambivalence could include a person's expression that "exercise will help me lose weight," but may also hold the view that "physical activity is painful and time consuming." In addition to the previously stated description of MI, motivational interviewing also decreases clients' resistance to change and increases change talk. Some examples of change talk include, but are not limited to, desire, ability, reasons, need, and commitment. Additionally, motivational interviewing can help an individual recognize the discrepancy between the desire to work out more frequently and lose weight and their actions, or lack thereof, with regard to obtaining their desired goals.

After learning both evidence-based motivational and behavioral change tools, you will be on your way to behavioral change as it pertains to engaging in regular physical activity. Along the way to mastering these tools to get you hooked on exercise, you will learn the program's weekly regimen of strength training and cardio. A lot of fitness plans or weight loss plans are difficult to follow for most people's lifestyles. The fitness regimens in this program are not easy; however, they were designed to prevent burn out by mixing up the work out and keeping them realistic, balanced, and doable for your busy daily life.

The passion for working out is what this program will give you and by continuing to utilize the information provided in this book, you will be able to tap into your newly found or regained passion to ignite your fitness motivation. This program is intended to show you that the little bit of pain you feel will turn into the fix that you crave. Keep in mind that, as a product of your efforts in this program, your mind and body will transform for the better.

You are now ready to say goodbye to your "before" body and your "before" beliefs, attitudes, and behaviors. The rest of this book will teach you how to enhance your self-control, empowerment, and motivation to actively engage in *your* life on your way toward fitness success.

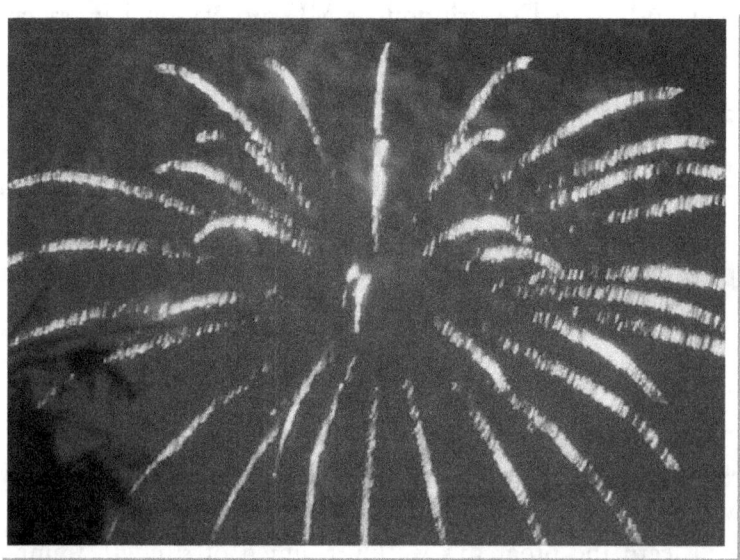

Chapter Two

THE MIND-BODY EFFECTS OF WORKING-OUT

Establishing the habit of exercising regularly will be one of the most important habits you will create in your life. Engaging in physical activity immediately increases levels of dopamine that helps exercise become a self-reinforcing behavior. If you continue on your fitness regimen consistently, and stay with your schedule for the most part, your brain cells in the motivation center of the brain will create new dopamine receptors. As a result, exercise will become a self-reinforcing behavior and you will gain the self-motivation that is essential in staying with a fitness regimen for life.

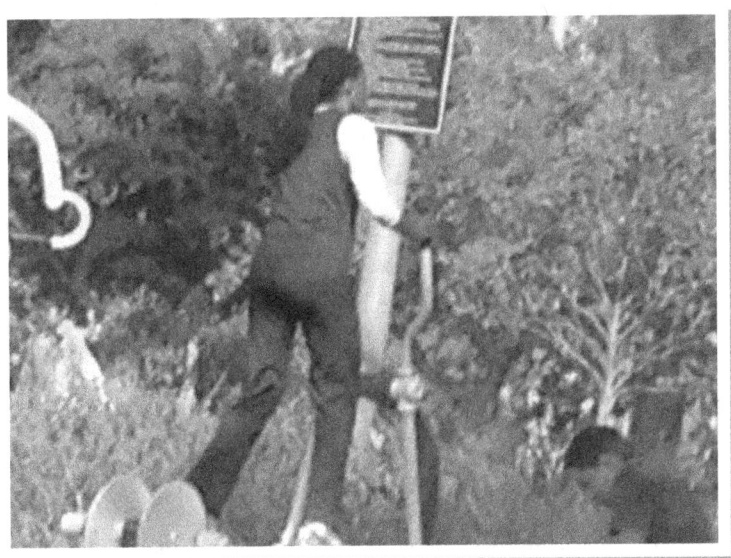

Depression and Exercise

Every year, Major Depressive Disorder negatively affects millions of American adults. Research for depressive issues and physical activity shows that the mental and physical gains of exercise can greatly help improve mood. Moreover, research shows that releasing feel-good neurochemicals, such as endorphins, as a product of physical fitness activity causes a feeling of wellness for body and mind. Physical fitness engagement helps greatly improve mood as well as energy and might help reduce depressive symptoms.

Despite the fact that regular physical activity may help relieve depression, only a small percentage of Americans participate in fitness activity at the recommended level As a result, many American adults don't engage in regular fitness activity and thus do not benefit from the positive mental health effects of exercise.

Although exercise can be beneficial to the mental health of clients, many depressed individuals do not engage in enough physical activity and, therefore, are not able to benefit from the mood-elevating effects caused by regular exercise. Depressed individuals often struggle to maintain the motivation necessary to participate in regular physical activity. Although working out may be beneficial to the mental health of clients, it is difficult for most individuals to comply with a physical activity regimen. However, making changes to one's behavior (such as engaging in physical activity) can lead to a significant improvement in mood and overall well-being.

Depression affects more millions of people globally. The lifetime risk for Major Depressive Disorder (MDD) has varied from 5 to 12 percent for adult men and 10 to 25 percent for adult women. Moreover, research suggests that people with depression are at more prone to chronic medical conditions and a higher rate of early death. Individuals with depression as well as other severe mental illnesses report worse general health and lack of exercise in their daily lives.

Currently, doctors in Britain recommend exercise first in their treatment of patients with depressive issues. However, this recommended treatment of physical activity is significantly underutilized in the United States. In addition, there's been a remarkably unfortunate increase in sedentary lifestyles from the increase in television viewing, *resulting in a large percent of adults engaging in no physical activity whatsoever*. It's no wonder why obesity is still number two when it comes to deaths that are preventable in the United States.

Many diseases, diabetes, some cancers, and depression are associated with excess weight and obesity. The individuals who experience depressive symptoms are not typically likely to participate in regular in fitness regimens. Additionally, the inverse relationship between fitness engagement and depressive symptoms has been extensively researched. Unfortunately, a lack of exercise participation has been associated with increased risk for depression.

Exercise has been shown to alleviate symptoms of depressive disorder when used as the only form of treatment. Moreover, most research shows the mood-enhancing effect of physical fitness activity is incredibly similar to traditional psychotherapy as well as psychiatric medications for depression. Combining psychiatric medications with exercise can then, in theory, have a more rapid effect on mood due to the accelerated effect of anti-depressant action (which would be beneficial considering that medications typically take several weeks to take effect). Also, exercise is a valid treatment strategy for major depressive disorder due to the fact that remaining on an exercise intervention could, in theory, be as effective as remaining on a psychiatric medications. Overall, this means that exercising along with taking antidepressants would speed up the positive mood effect and that people are likely to adhere just as much, if not more, to an exercise regimen as they would a medication regimen.

Developing a healthy lifestyle that includes physical activity is an integral part of mental well-being that is not commonly looked at in mental health treatment settings. Though upping levels of exercise can result in reducing depressive symptoms, feeling fatigued and experiencing low energy could prevent individuals with depressive disorders from remaining on fitness regimens including voluntary fitness. Empirical evidence suggests that adults, including women experiencing menopausal symptoms, can reduce their depressive symptoms and increase positive affects with physical activities such as cardiorespiratory fitness. Despite barriers such as depressed mood, fatigue, low energy, and diminished interest in activities, exercise can be beneficial to depressed individuals and may be utilized as part of a treatment program designed to enhance self-esteem and mood.

Psychological and Physiological Effects of Exercise on Mood

Several neurobiological systems may be working when clients report that physical activity helps them feel less depressed. The popular term of the Neuro-chemical benefit of exercise is the "runner's high," that is the sense of analgesia (pain insensitivity) as well as euphoria felt after intense exercise. Endorphins are stress hormones that relieve muscle pain and calm the brain during strenuous exercise. Moreover, endorphins produced in the brain are known to contribute to the feeling of well-being that typically comes along with exercise. Due to the fact that plasma levels of opioids increase as a result of exercise, these opioids most likely play a role in improved mood after exercise. Thus, the endogenous opioids known as endorphins are known to be the cause of the "runner's high" phenomenon.

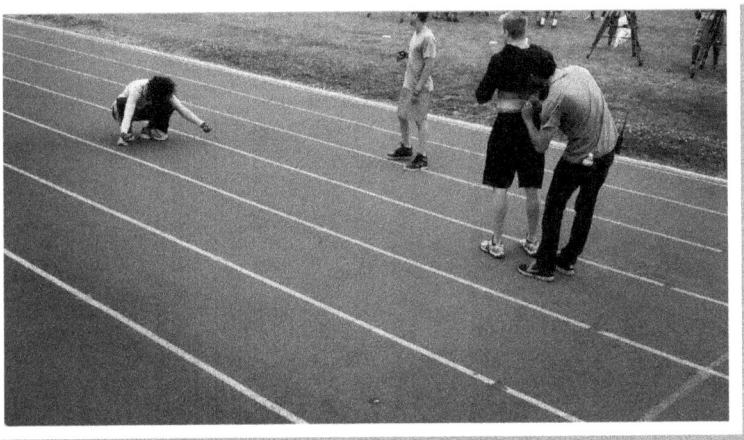

Another neurobiological system that may contribute to mood enhancement is the monoamine mechanism. Monoamines are involved in depression and many antidepressant medications increase the amounts of monoamines. Examples of monoamines include dopamine, epinephrine, serotonin, and norepinephrine. It is hypothesized that physical activity may stimulate production of monoamines. One particular monoamine, known as dopamine, plays a significant role in motivation and attention. When a person engages in physical activity, dopamine levels are increased in the brain, which results in feelings of well-being, accomplishment, and overall mood improvement. Chronic exercise increases dopamine storage in the brain and promotes the production of enzymes that form dopamine receptors in the reward center of the brain.

Physical activity regulates every one of the neurotransmitters targeted by antidepressants. Research studies showing that physical activity increases the available amount of norepinephrine as well as serotonin create interest due to the fact that most antidepressant medications, including tricyclics, SSRIs, norepinephrine and serotonin reuptake inhibitors, and MAOIs, increase norepinephrine and/or serotonin levels. Exercise immediately elevates levels of norepinephrine in the brain. In addition, serotonin is similarly affected by exercise and it plays a significant role in self-esteem, impulse control, and mood improvement. Although research suggests the factor of monoamines in major depressive disorder and great benefits of physical activity for mood, researchers have recently become aware of the problems arising out of the monoamine hypothesis with regard to depression. Among about one-third of individuals struggling with major depressive disorder, a significant portion of the already available psychiatric medications used to treat depression do not seem to be work in treating their depressive issues.

Systematic studies have been done on the most effective way of dealing with depressive symptoms that negatively affect individuals' ability to participate and benefit from physical activity. Strategies to improve physical activity participation levels that have been effective in healthy individuals can be used for those struggling with depression.

Exercise Effects on Mind and Body Simplified:

Working out affects the brain and the entire body. Since your heart is really a muscle (and responds to fitness as other muscles) it becomes larger and strengthens with regular exercise. When your heart is stronger it is more efficient. Aerobic exercise is greatly beneficial for the heart and it helps you to build endurance. In addition to getting in cardio, it is essential that you add weight training to your fitness routine. Weight training builds your muscles, which helps burn body fat, and as an added bonus it helps improve bone density. Fitness participation helps strengthen the skeletal system through bone building via osteoblast cell activation. Both resistance exercise and weight lifting can improve bone density. Exercise also helps to improve healthy levels of one's cholesterol. Blood pressure levels can also be helped through moderate forms of exercise. Moderate exercise gives an overall boost to the immune system.

When it comes to the brain, exercise helps to activate neurotransmitters (as we discussed previously). These neurotrasmitters are "feel good" chemicals in the brain that are released when you exercise. They include dopamine, norepinephrine; acetylcholine, and serotonin, which helps you to calm and to sleep. When it comes to aging, it has been shown that women who are physically active experience less mental decline as compared to the women who refrain from engaging in regular physical activity. Therefore, regular exercise results in a better mind and a better body.

"Working-Out" Your Stress

Some of the most effective people I have met work physical activity into their routine almost every day. From speakers and authors, to actors and business owners, the successful individuals that I know choose to manage their daily stress by working out on a regular basis. They make a conscious decision and an ongoing dedication, not simply despite their busy schedules, *but because of their busy schedules*. These highly successful and effective people continue with their active lifestyles for the purpose of maintaining the energy to sustain the highest level of performance in all areas of their lives. As a result, they benefit personally, socially, sexually, and occupationally which translates into overall life satisfaction.

Situations that have the potential to cause stress (whether socially, physically, or occupationally) are an inevitable part of life. Despite the fact that you may not have the option of preventing the situation, you do hold the option to control your psychological and physiological stress levels. When stress goes untreated for long periods of time it turns into chronic stress. Chronic stress is toxic to the mind and body and has the potential to result in physical disease (such as cancer, high blood pressure, and heart problems) and mental disorders (such as anxiety disorder and depressive disorder).

Negative moods are associated with high levels of stress. A relevant mechanism for exercise-associated mood changes is called the HPA axis which is responsible for controlling your reactions to stress. The HPA axis plays a major role in depression and stress response. It regulates response in the body (caused by stress) by releasing numerous stress hormones. Additionally, the HPA axis is known to function abnormally in individuals with major depression. In response to physical (exercise) and psychological stress, stress hormones are released by the HPA axis. Although over-training increases stress hormone release, moderate training decreases the stress hormone release. Additionally, long-term participation in physical activity seems effective in minimizing a body's response to stress in the body caused by exercise as well as overall stress.

Therefore, in addition to the previously discussed mechanisms for exercise-associated mood changes, the HPA axis may also play a role in mood enhancement.

Improvements in Mood and Self-Worth

Depression can result from feeling helpless and believing that there is nothing one can do to improve one's mood and/or situation. Exercise can often provide a sense of mastery and control. Low self-efficacy (the sense of being able to take control of one's life) worsens outcomes in depression. However, engagement in fitness routines has been shown to improve an individual's ability to take back control of one's life. As a result, physical activity may be an effective way for a client to feel a sense of control in his/her life. A sense of control can result in a sense of mastery, which can lead to increased self-esteem, and exercise has the potential to alleviate depression due to self-esteem enhancement. Lastly, improvement in mood may also increase the potential for a person to continue working-out due to the positive effect on self-esteem.

Recommended Guidelines for Physical Activity

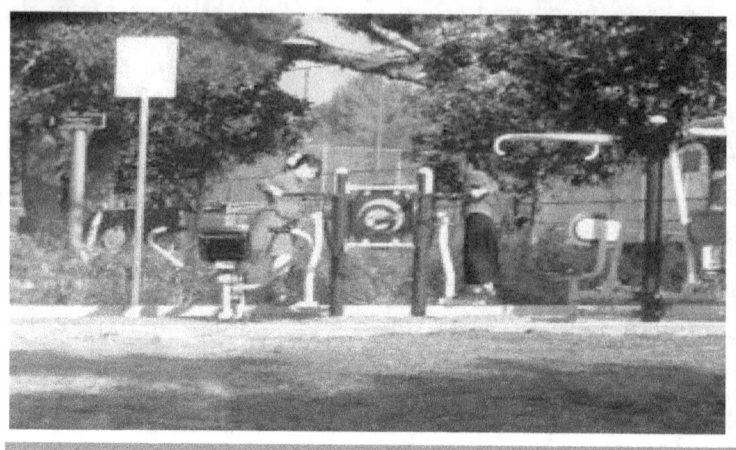

A recommendation for exercise to almost every individual is unlikely to cause harm and likely to be very beneficial. In the past, what was recommended for exercise was thirty minutes of physical fitness activity (moderate intensity) for the majority of the days of the week. Currently, the weekly recommendation for physical activity (for individuals aged 18 to 65) is two and a half hours of cardio (moderate intensity) in addition to muscle strengthening (such as resistance training or weight lifting) on two or more days. Exercise and mixed exercise (aerobic and resistance) are more effective than aerobic exercise alone in reducing patient-perceived symptoms of depression.

Another notable form of exercise that has been proven to reduce symptoms of depression is "mindful" exercise. Examples of mindful exercises include Tai Chi and yoga. Studies involving adults report very significant mental and physical effects from lifestyle intervention programs that focus on mind and body exercises Tai Chi and yoga.

Walking is the number one (as far as frequency) recommended form of physical fitness activity within health care settings. Moreover, walking may be more adhered to than other exercises.

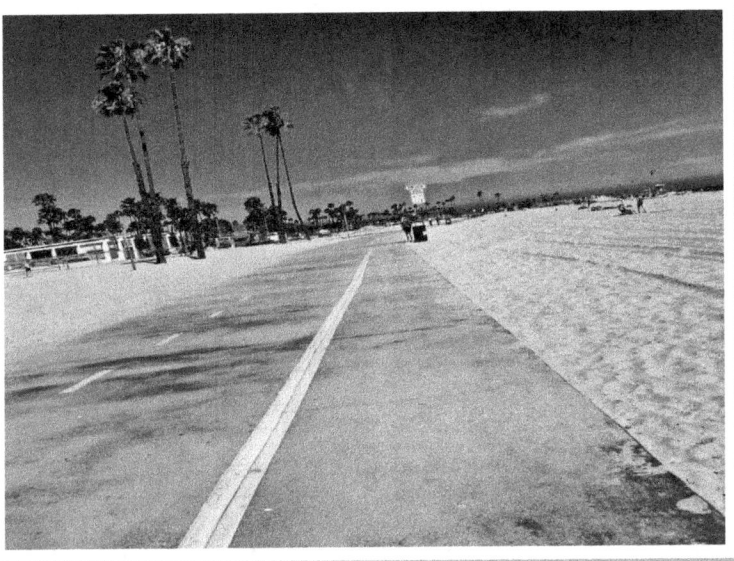

Although walking is known as the most frequent form of physical activity recommended by health care professionals, mixed exercise (aerobic and resistance) is more effective than aerobic exercise alone in reducing patient-perceived symptoms of depression. In health care settings, advice from a medical professional has the potential to lead to short-term (less than 12 weeks) increases in physical activity. However, referrals to exercise specialists can lead to long-term (up to eight months) change in both health care and community settings. It is critical for all individuals that have risk factors for cardiovascular disease to seek a medical clearance prior to participating in a fitness activity regimen.

Routine and Consistency Equals Success

No matter the form of exercise you choose (the one recommended to you in this book, or a physical hobby, or a combination thereof) the key to making your motivation last and maintaining your ideal body is CONSISTENCY!

Set the amount of days you will be active and stick to your routine. The fitness regimen that will fit into your schedule is the one you will embrace and be able to continue in the long-term.

Research shows that approximately half of those who begin a new fitness regimen drop out within six months to a year. *One of the major reasons why people fail to keep up with their fitness regimens is that they begin a workout that is not appropriate for their fitness level.* As a result, they feel that they are not good enough to stick with the work out and they quit. You may have experienced an intense workout that made you vomit afterwards (literally) and left you feeling defeated. Remember, when you begin my workout regimen (later in the book) that it is more important to do some of the workout consistently than nothing or sometimes. I have had many clients who (despite not being in the mood and having busy schedules) made sure they did at least part of their workout when it was scheduled.

Establishing the habit of exercising regularly (even if it is some of the workout and you remain on schedule) will be among the most essential habits you will create for yourself. Since engaging in exercise immediately increases levels of dopamine, exercise will become a self-reinforcing behavior for you. When you continue on your fitness regimen on a consistent basis, and stay with your schedule for the most part, your brain cells in the motivation center of the brain will create new dopamine receptors. As a result, you will gain the self-motivation that is essential in staying with a fitness routine for life.

You can use the techniques in this program to have fitness motivation for life. You will also accomplish something more powerful: you will prove to yourself that you have the power to change your thoughts and behaviors and improve your mood. This power will increase your confidence and you will view yourself in a new and incredible way. You will also empower yourself with the tools that will help you achieve greater control of your mind, body, and quality of life.

Chapter Three

"Working Out" Your Intentions

Desire is the beginning phase of achievement! You have longed for a better body, more energy, and an overall sense of confidence and achievement. Such longing has undoubtedly brought you to this point of acquiring the tools to help these goals manifest. Longing is simply not enough. In order for you to take the next step, you must create focused and powerful thoughts and feelings that will lead you to your physical transformation.

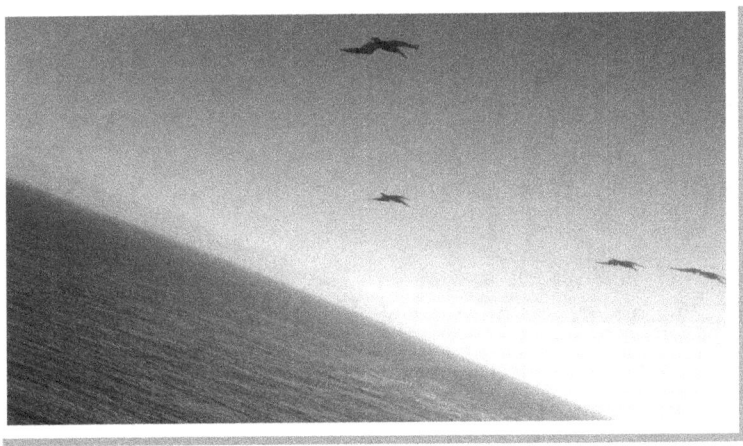

The Science behind Intending a Better Body

"I admit that thoughts influence the body." – Albert Einstein

Neuroscientists have come up with a system that analyses activity in the brain to work out an individual's intentions prior to them having executed the behavior. A team of leading neuroscientists has developed a way to analyze the brain for information about intentions that would not be able to be seen from the outside. They conducted a study to measure intentions before a person acts using a scanner. This advance in research proves that intentions are very real-real enough to be analyzed by technology. Intentions can be used to help manifest a better body, more energy, and overall well-being.

Create the Intention

You may be stuck as a result of negative thinking and a lack of intending the results you desire.

Are your thoughts getting in your way?

You can learn to work through doubt, fear, worry, and other such negative self-talk to create confidence and a healthy self-image before actually attaining your better body. Similar to goals you have accomplished in your past, the **pulsating intention** is everything when it comes to attaining your goals for the near future.

First Steps:

1. Gain clarity about what it is you want and write it.

2. Share your intention: talk about the intention with someone supportive who will help you be accountable.

3. Commit to your intention by taking some action today.

4. Continue to feel strongly positive about your intention (use positive affirmations to help you stay positive such as "I deserve to be healthy and happy", "I am making

room for all the good I want to come into my life,"and "I'm deserving and grateful and I accept this change."

It is critical that you become clear about what you are intending into your life. One powerful way to help you create the **pulsating intention** to have more energy and be more fit is through meditation. Meditation is a technique used to promote relaxation and awareness. You may put yourself into a very relaxed state of mind (with or without relaxing music) and implant your new intention by concentrating on it for at least sixty seconds. The meditation does not need to be complicated. You can engage in the practice by simply deep breathing (and progressive muscle relaxation if you choose) and focusing on your intention for a few minutes.

While meditating, imagine your intention vividly, so in your mind's eye, picture what your life will be like once the intention has already manifested (i.e. once you are living in your new and energized body). Inject a great deal of positive emotion into these visualizations as well. If you can't create strong positive emotions, then you will not be able to create your **pulsating intention**. If you must, you may alter the intention to make it seem more believable for you. Your intention must have the pulsating desire behind it to manifest. You must really, really, really want it, intend it powerfully through meditation, intend strongly with positive emotions, and continue all of your energy and dedication going forward to allow the intention to become your new reality.

At first, you may be frustrated because you feel as if you cannot seem to focus for a enough of a length of time. You may keep falling back into previous ways of thinking even without trying and thus squash your most important intentions in just days, or even hours. Killing your good intentions results in a lack of manifestation. If you aren't content with the way your mind and body is now: intend change. Know that what you think about intently can result in attainment of results and we all wants results!

Thoughts control decisions which end up controlling results. When understood, you can begin to assume a great level of respect for your thoughts. You can decide to obtain control of your own thoughts. You may see that you are unwilling to simply accept what you don't want (like an out of shape body). It is important to develop an apparent and lasting respect for the power that intention has for your life.

As you are achieving your desires faster than ever before, you may feel inclined to engage in more and more thinking, feeling, acting, as well as meditating in a manner that is aligned with your goals. It is recommended that you spend about thirty or so minutes per day holding intentions with positive feelings and allowing them to circle around and marinade in your imagination. You can do what feels most natural to you to manifest your goals with your pulsating intention. Enjoy as your thoughts, feelings, actions, and physical body begin to align with your pulsating intentions.

Your goal to lose weight, or become toned, or have more energy, or look sexier starts by setting an intention. Your intention will help you in gaining greater control over your own life. An intention is essentially having a plan as well as a purpose to focus the mind and go for the goal. According to cognitive behavioral therapy (CBT), thoughts control feelings which control behaviors. In a later chapter in this book, you will be able to use CBT interventions focused on interventions to:

▶ Identify the unconscious intentions that guide your cognitive process, belief system, and behavior

- ▶ By becoming mindful of the intentions behind much of your negative thoughts, feelings, and actions, you can accept control, and begin the process of mind and body change

- ▶ Notice how you have created your body and life as it is presently through conscious and unconscious intention

- ▶ Live intentionally through focused, open, non-judging, acceptance of yourself

- ▶ Create your life consciously in the way that is most fulfilling and desirable for you

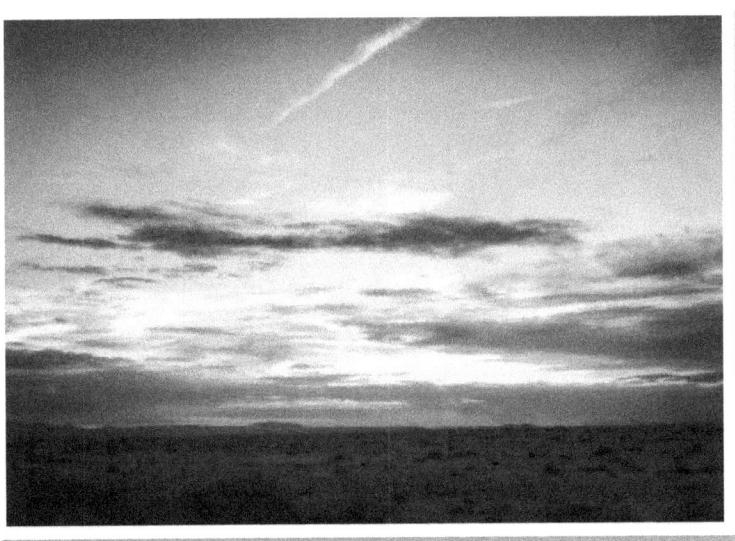

The Take-Home about Intentions

An intention is not something you set and lose track of, rather, it is something you hold onto strongly, think and feel positively about, of which you allow your actions and eventual reality to transpire. Remember to take powerful, informed (which you are because you are reading this right now), deliberate actions to make your dreams a reality. It is your time to create your new reality. You have the ability and potential to achieve health and happiness and the body you have always desired. Keep going and don't give up!

Your pulsating intention can transform the conversation around your goals from impossible to possible. An intention mixed with strong positive thoughts and feelings (which is what makes the intention pulsate) will align your behaviors with your desired goal.

What will you intend?

PART II

Altering Fitness-Related Thoughts and Behaviors

Chapter Four

CHANGING THE IRRATIONAL BELIEFS THAT KEEP YOU UNFIT

Turn your dreams into plans!

What do you think would happen if you replaced an irrational belief such as, "I won't ever be fit because all I've ever been is out of shape" or, "I'm not disciplined enough to meet my fitness goals" with the positive affirmation quote at the beginning of this chapter? If you are pessimistic about yourself and/or your ability to change, you are most likely up against irrational beliefs. Irrational beliefs must be acknowledged as irrational before you take even one more step in this mind and body transformation. The reason for this is simply that, if you embark on your fitness program before ridding yourself of your irrational beliefs, you may eventually self-sabotage because you don't believe you are capable of attaining or deserving of the results.

Irrational beliefs are self-inflicted negative beliefs. They keep us from attaining our personal and professional goals. They stop us from accomplishing our goals and often times limit us from our true potential. These irrational beliefs most likely are unproductive, unrealistic expectations exacted on ourselves that often result in continuing negative self-concepts and unrealized goals. In order to realize your goals, it is paramount that we rid ourselves of irrational beliefs by challenging them and affirming our new more positive beliefs.

Examples that Represent Irrational Beliefs

Irrational beliefs about oneself:

▶ If I can't do the exercise fully, I might as well not try

▶ I've always failed at my weight loss goals so why try now

▶ I don't deserve good attention from others

▶ I'm lazy

▶ I am too weak to attempt a fitness program

▶ I am not worth the effort

▶ I'm not an athlete and never will be

▶ I will never be fit, it's just not in my genes

▶ I'm not disciplined enough

▶ I am an unattractive fat person so it doesn't even matter

▶ I will always be out of shape no matter how hard I try

▶ There is only one way and I can't do it

▶ There is only black/white and right/wrong (this is dichotomous thinking that sets a person up for failure)

Research shows that irrational beliefs may interfere with a person's participation in physical activity. The following are additional examples of irrational beliefs: (a) "If I don't workout to full capacity I'm a failure"; (b) "I must exercise at the highest level to gain people's approval, and if not then I'm not good enough"; "The aspects of my life must work out with regard to getting what I want now easily (such as rapid weight loss)." These types of irrational beliefs can deter you from your goals and prevent you from living your ideal life. You may have an irrational belief of your own that is preventing you from ultimate success. Distorted thinking such as catastrophizing and believing that their self-worth depends on achievement can have devastating effects on one's performance.

People are often unaware of their distorted thinking patterns. They are also unaware of how these irrational beliefs can result in sub-par levels of energy, lack of motivation, and difficulty in engaging in exercise due to self-doubt. Identifying these distortions is critical adapting a rational way of thinking that directly affects one's ability to participate actively in life. Identification of distorted thinking can be done through writing in a journal or engagement of physical activity while verbalizing positive affirmations in the presence of a mental health professional. Toward the end of this chapter, I will provide for you tools that I would give a wellness coaching or therapy client to challenge their irrational beliefs and cognitive distortions for the purpose of increasing their motivation for positive change.

In a therapeutic setting, cognitive restructuring is implemented after the identification of irrational beliefs. Cognitive restructuring is an effective system for being able to recognize our thoughts and beliefs and altering these thoughts when they are no longer useful in our lives.

During the cognitive restructuring phase, a person realizes the inappropriateness of the current beliefs and positive beliefs are created. The restructuring may be accomplished by processing with clients to help them figure out whether the beliefs are helpful and whether or not their current beliefs help them reach their goals. Working out daily to create new positive associations in the brain) one learns that the experience can be enjoyable and can lead to rewards such as increased self-esteem and empowerment. Lastly, clients may benefit from using positive affirmations, such as "I want to be healthy and I have the ability to do so," "Exercise gives me the energy I need to live my life fully," and "I am doing my best and my self-worth does not depend on the approval of others."

Committing to Change for Life

We have a great ability to change our way of thinking for life. When you decide to change your irrational beliefs every day, by reaffirming your new positive beliefs and working on the exercises provided for you to use at the end of this chapter, you will find your thinking changing and becoming more aligned with the path toward your fitness and physical fitness goals. On the following page, you will find your "Fitness Motivation Toolbox" exercises. These exercises are customized for the purpose of establishing and maintaining the motivation to work out on a regular basis. All exercises are based on either cognitive behavioral therapy techniques or motivational interviewing techniques that are evidence-based techniques. The truth is that you are tomorrow what you establish today. You are on your way!

FITNESS MOTIVATION TOOLBOX

RECOGNIZING AND RIDDING OURSELVES OF IRRATIONAL BELIEFS

How to Recognize Irrational Beliefs:

Irrational beliefs are there when we:

- ▶ Are feeling paralyzed and unable to move forward in addressing our problems
- ▶ Find excuses to remain stuck
- ▶ Have been struggling with a problem for a great deal of time, however, we haven't taken enough steps to help ourselves
- ▶ Find we are remaining stuck by not even trying or self-sabotaging when we do try
- ▶ Find that we aren't able to make a centered decision

Benefits of Challenging Irrational Beliefs:

- ▶ Gain greater respect for ourselves
- ▶ Gain a better and more clear intention for our goals
- ▶ Eliminate or decrease the fear of taking on a new challenge
- ▶ Identify the obstacles that may come when starting on a new regimen
- ▶ Become solid and realistic about accomplishing our goals
- ▶ Feel productive even in times of distress
- ▶ Live more authentic and much more fulfilling lives
- ▶ View our lives in a more positive way
- ▶ Recognize our self-worth and potential
- ▶ Forgive the mistakes we have made
- ▶ Give ourselves understanding and encouragement

FITNESS MOTIVATION TOOLBOX

IDENTIFYING IRRATIONAL BELIEFS

Even if you feel that you have no irrational beliefs, dig deep, and try to find any beliefs that may lie in your conscious or subconscious mind that have previously prevented you from achieving your goals. Are you able to state the irrational belief or beliefs? If yes, write them down in your journal:

"My beliefs that are blocking me from my goals are..."

_____

_____

_____

_____

_____

_____

_____

_____

_____

_____

FITNESS MOTIVATION TOOLBOX

QUESTIONS TO ASK YOURSELF ABOUT IRRATIONAL BELIEFS

Since you have identified these irrational belief/beliefs, the next step is to try to identify how it is blocking you from obtaining your goals. Answer these questions in your journal.

1. Is the belief a belief that I've believed in all my life?

_____

2. Where did I originally obtain this belief?

_____

_____

_____

3. Did this belief used to serve me in the past?

_____

_____

4. Is the belief still serving me or is it no longer useful?

_____

5. Does the belief make me feel defeated? _____

6. Is the belief keeping me stuck and triggering fear of guilt as I confront this problem?

_____

_____

7. Is the belief a feeling or an intuition? _____

Once you have identified the belief and asked yourself the previous questions, the next step is to test its accuracy. The following questions are regarding the belief... answer either "yes" or "no."

1. Is there proof in to support the belief as *always* being true?
_____

2. Does your belief aid with personal growth, positive behavior change and consistent motivation? _____

3. If you stick with this belief, will it help you to overcome obstacles in your personal or professional life? _____

4. Does this belief cause behavior that's self-defeating?
_____

5. Does this belief stop you from making wise decisions?
_____

6. Does this belief negatively affect your ability to resolve problems resulting in feeling paralyzed? _____

7. Is this a yes or no, black or white, all or nothing type of belief? _____

If you found yourself answering **no** to one or more of questions 1 through 3 and **yes** to most answers 4 through 7, then your belief is most likely irrational.

FITNESS MOTIVATION TOOLBOX

CHALLENGING YOUR IRRATIONAL BELIEFS

Once you have discovered whether your beliefs are irrational, you are prepared to challenge the beliefs. Answer these questions in your journal for each of your irrational beliefs (or choose one that is getting in your way most):

1. What is the feeling I get most of the time when I think about this belief?

_____

_____

2. Is there something in reality to support that the belief is completely true?

_____

3. What in the real world supports what's untrue in this belief?

_____

4. What's the worst outcome that could happen if I let go of this belief?

_____

_____

5. What positive outcomes could happen if I let go of this belief?

_____

_____

_____

6. What would be a realistic and appropriate belief I could swap out for this irrational belief?

_____

_____

_____

_____

_____

7. How could I grow if I replace the irrational belief for the positive and rational belief?

_____

_____

_____

_____

_____

8. What is preventing me from accepting the new replacement positive belief?

_____

_____

_____

Now that you have answered the previous questions, substitute your irrational belief/beliefs for positive and more rational beliefs. Then take action:

"My replacement and new rational belief/beliefs is/are…"

_____

_____

_____

_____

_____

_____

_____

_____

_____

_____

_____

_____

_____

_____

_____

_____

_____

FITNESS MOTIVATION TOOLBOX

FROM IRRATIONAL TO RATIONAL BELIEFS WITH POSITIVE AFFIRMATIONS

Research shows that positive affirmations are powerful life changers. The following affirmations can be repeated daily until you internalize them and truly *believe* them. It may be beneficial to write these down and post them places (in your home, car, office, or in your social media) where you will see them on a regular basis. Enjoy!

► My tomorrow depends on what I establish today.

► I am a strong person.

► I'm healthy and very happy.

► I am an athlete.

► My body is in good condition and I can accomplish my fitness goals.

► I have plenty of energy to work out.

► My body and mind are energetic.

► I can work out regularly.

► I have so much vitality.

► I feel good in all aspects of my being.

► I can always do at least some of my work out if not all.

► I am filled with hope

► My behaviors match my new positive beliefs

► My thoughts are focused on my fitness goals.

► I deserve a lean healthy body and I'm ready for it.

► I can already see myself looking and feeling better.

FITNESS MOTIVATION TOOLBOX

FINAL WORKSHEET: MOTIVATIONAL WORDS FOR YOUR NEW RATIONAL BELIEFS

Due to numerous influences, we take on our thinking styles, both irrational and rational. You may be recognizing some of your irrational beliefs, however, you may still ask, "How and why do I think that way?" The truth is you are halfway there and may have not even realized it. Most of the benefits come from recognizing the irrational beliefs are not helpful for you. The next step, however, is the one which requires more applied work and that is challenging the negative thinking, habitually and often. You will able to accomplish your goals much more effectively by establishing rational beliefs that are positive and aligned with achievement with the tools already provided for you.

Your brain may not immediately feel very comfortable at the beginning with a new type of thinking similar to your body not feeling comfortable immediately learning a new task. The more you practice, however, the more it will become automatic.

Chapter Five

MOTIVATIONAL INTERVIEWING FOR EXERCISE MOTIVATION

What kind of results do you want? Many of us want the fire under us that makes us want to work out and sustain a routine that gets the results. Since you are reading this book, you understand that it takes programming your mind at a deeper level (deeper than the hype of a New Year's resolution) in order to stay on a fitness routine. In fact, research by the University of Hertfordshire shows that people who made a two-week resolution failed before the half-way stage. *This means that many people burn out after a mere week after making a New Year's resolution.* The results of this remarkable study also demonstrated that people who use techniques rather than will-power alone are able to continue their resolutions for a longer period of time.

An optimal technique that is supported by the research for exercise motivation is motivational interviewing (MI). When you are seeking the motivation to gain results (for a better body, sharper mind, etc. from regular exercise) motivational interviewing falls into the "what you need" category to get you "what you want"...*results.*

MI has been shown to be enhanced when MI is combined with other effective treatment methods such as cognitive behavioral therapy (which was discussed in the previous chapter). The technique of motivational interviewing can be used to improve a person's motivation to change and it can be effective in facilitating behavioral change.

In a clinical setting, motivational interviewing is used by a therapist or other mental health or medical professional to help promote positive change in a client's behavior. MI exercises are designed to help people recognize the need for changes in their behavior. As a first exercise, let's say a motivational interviewer (i.e. psychologists, nurses, social workers, medical practitioners, physiotherapists, and dietitians) is meeting with a client trying to lose weight to alleviate chronic health problems. The motivational interviewer would emphasize the importance of the change, current information about why the client should make the alteration in his/her lifestyle, including many benefits. The motivational interviewer would then provide the steps and action plan to make these lifestyle changes. At the end of this chapter, you will be given tools based on the technique of motivational interviewing to help you in your personal fitness goals.

Motivational interviewing is an evidence-based technique that is proven to help even depressed individuals increase their motivation to work out. People with depression often lack the motivation necessary to change their behaviors. Depression makes it difficult for people to begin, or adhere to, recommendations given to them by mental health professionals. In addition, depression can contribute to an individual's lack of motivation due to such factors as being in a depressive mood, lost interest in most of their typical activities, and lower than normal energy levels. As a result, depressed clients are not as likely to remain engaging in healthy behaviors, such as fitness routines.

Motivational interviewing is a client-centered technique used to enhance motivation that comes from within to increase healthy behaviors by processing and resolving ambivalence. Ambivalence is the conflict individuals experience when exploring the costs and benefits of engaging in a particular behavior. An example of ambivalence could include a client's expression that "exercise will help me lose weight" but may also hold the view that "physical activity is painful and time consuming." In addition to the previously stated description of MI, motivational interviewing also decreases clients' resistance to change and increases change talk. Some examples of change talk include but are not limited to desire, ability, reasons, need, and commitment. Additionally, motivational interviewing can help the client recognize the discrepancy between their desires and their actions, or lack thereof, with regard to obtaining their desired goals.

In the beginning phase of therapy, the therapist concentrates on promoting self-talk for the purpose of increasing intrinsic motivation to alter behavior. In this case, the behavioral change would be to increase physical activity. A typical first session would begin with the therapist asking the client open-ended questions to elicit change self-talk. Then, the mental health professional asserts feedback/response from the client's original session. Finally, toward the latter end of the assessment, the mental health professional collaborates with the client to develop a change plan (if the client asserts his willingness to change) and asks the client for commitment. When significant motivation appears to be apparent in the client, the mental health professional goes into the next phase of commitment to change. During this phase, the sessions focus transitioning from motivation into commitment with focus on specific change plans including goals and implementation.

The transcript that follows is a transcript that illustrates the use of motivational interviewing for the purpose of motivating a client to engage in physical activity:

THERAPIST: "We've talked about a lot, and you're developing a nice list of things you can do to make your life more fulfilling, longer, and happier. Is there anything else from that list I gave you earlier that you'd like to talk about?"

PATIENT: "Maybe nutrition and exercise."

THERAPIST: "What are your concerns in this area?"

PATIENT: "I'm not concerned really. I'm just wondering what I should be doing."

THERAPIST: "There are quite a lot of things you could do such as making incremental, gradual changes in your activity levels and building some modest exercise into your regular routine. Would this be workable for you?"

PATIENT: "Well maybe, but I would rather not get a gym membership or anything like that. I really don't need another heart attack."

THERAPIST: "Adding some kind of exercise will be okay for you, but definitely not the gym yet. What kind of physical activity do you get at the moment?"

PATIENT: "Not much. I just do a bit of dog walking a few times a week. Sometimes when walking him I get these feelings in my chest and I worry I'm pushing too hard."

THERAPIST: "That is a common worry, and our experience suggests that as long as you things gradually, no harm should come your way. We could work together to help you develop a gradual program to increase your activity levels. If you'd prefer, you could even use the facilities here, and we can monitor your heart rate to make sure it's safe."

PATIENT: "That sounds really good. Mostly I think walking is what will work for me. I could do more of that especially around the park near my house."

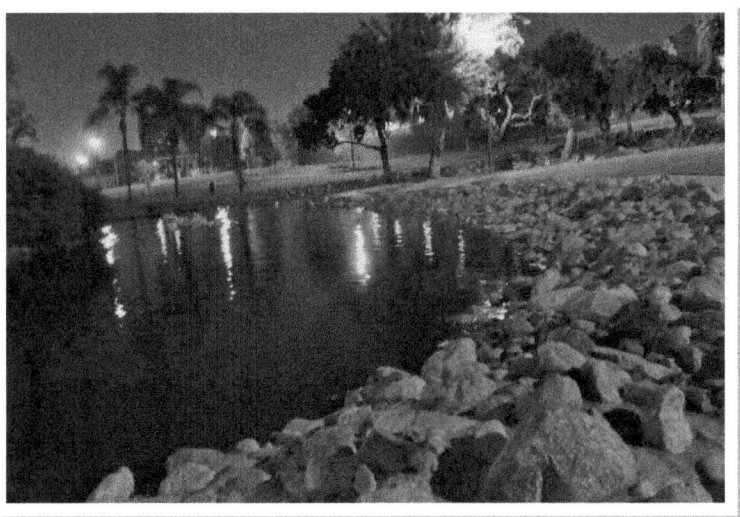

THERAPIST: "That's what's important-to find what you like to do that works for you and fits with your normal life.

PATIENT: "Okay. I'll take you up on a little monitoring while I exercise here as well. That sounds like it will work for me."

Motivational interviewing has been effectively used in numerous studies that analyzed significant changes of lifestyle behaviors, such as exercise participation. MI has been indicated in research to be effective in both decreasing maladaptive behaviors and in promoting adaptive behaviors, such as exercise. While implementing MI, therapists promote a client's personal form of motivation rather than attempting to install a kind of motivation as it is important that individuals realize that self-empowerment is critical for maintaining behavioral change.

When setting goals for yourself, it is helpful to use the acronym SMART which is *specific*, easy to *measure*, quite *achievable*, definitely *realistic*, and must be *timely*. There are several tools used by health professionals for motivational interviewing. A decisional balance sheet that lists the pros and cons for exercising or not exercising can be utilized. You will be very able to complete this exercise toward the end of this chapter. Additionally, individuals can use a scale in which confidence can be measured. On this scale they rate their confidence with regard to ability to execute the action plan on a scale from zero to ten. In the case that you rate lower than seven, your need for improving confidence should be identified and processed. Moreover, you can utilize psycho-education as a motivational tool. This means that you research all of the benefits of exercise such as those outlined in the beginning of this book.

According to the research, messages for motivation in printed form (or on a computer document) appear to be significantly more effective than face-to-face talk therapy alone when it comes to clients being motivated for change. These motivational tools can all be utilized to contribute to your lifestyle modification program and they are provided for you toward the end of the chapter.

According to the research, it is important that individuals adhere to the following guidelines when translating intrinsic motivation into practical physical activity promotion. One, you should *emphasize individual mastery*. Two, *perceptions of choice, fun and the excitement of exercise should be promoted.*

Third, it is important to *promote a sense of purpose by learning the value of exercise to health, optimal function, and overall quality of life.*

You should avoid turning exercise into a chore. It is also important that you give yourself encouragement along the way and surround yourself with supportive company as research shows that people who are provided with positive feedback tend to have higher intrinsic motivation in comparison with those not rewarded.

We know interventions that promote physical activity are of great value, as engaging in regular exercise may help individuals in areas such as overall physical health, self-esteem, stress reduction, and mood enhancement. Cognitive behavioral therapy and motivational interviewing are interventions that can help empower depressed clients to engage in long-term physical activity, therefore improving their quality of life.

By focusing on your future, rather than past failures, and by practicing these types of interventions, you can trigger confidence in adopting new patterns in dealing with difficult times. As a result, you can move toward long-term staying with healthy behaviors, such as engaging in a regular fitness regimen.

DECISIONS FOR CHANGE WORKSHEET

When we consider changes we don't always consider the pros and cons of the situation. Thinking through the pros and cons of making this fitness-related change (as well as if we don't make the change) is a way to help us ensure we have thoroughly processed the prospect of the change. This can help us keep our plan even in stressful or challenging times.

	PROS/BENEFITS	CONS/COSTS
Making a Change		
Not Changing		

NEED FOR CHANGE ASSESSMENT

Think about something you want, need, or should be considering changing related to fitness. Ask yourself (in a mirror and then in writing) the following questions.

Why do I want to make a change?

_____

_____

_____

_____

How will I make this change?

_____

_____

_____

_____

_____

_____

_____

What are some reasons to make this change?

_____

_____

_____

_____

_____

_____

_____

_____

_____

_____

From one to ten (ten being the very most), how much do you want the results created by the change? _____

Rate your ability make the steps necessary to obtain your goals on a scale from 1 to 10. _____

(If you rate less than 7, your needs for improving confidence should be processed)

What is your *ideal* outcome if you decide to make this change?

CHANGE ACTION PLAN WORKSHEET

Setting Your Goals

Use specific, very measurable, appropriately achievable, realistic, and timely (SMART) and write down your goals.

The actual change I want to make in my life is:

_____

_____

_____

_____

_____

_____

The reasons for making this change are:

_____

_____

_____

_____

_____

The steps I will make for this change are:

_____

_____

_____

_____

_____

_____

_____

The ways others can help me are:

_____

_____

_____

_____

_____

_____

Some things that might get in the way of my plan are:

_____

_____

_____

_____

Some things I will do if I stop taking steps toward my goal are:

_____

_____

_____

_____

_____

I will know my plan is working and effective when:

_____

_____

_____

_____

_____

VISUALIZING THE FUTURE

This exercise is designed to help you develop skills in asking questions that prompt you to reflect on your current behavior and its impact it has on the future, write a letter (to yourself) as if it is a year from today. Write how successful you were in making the change, what changes you made, and how happy and proud you are that you made the change. Encourage yourself throughout the letter in order to provoke the stamina necessary to accomplish your goal.

_____

_____

_____

_____

_____

_____

_____

_____

_____

_____

_____

_____

Chapter Six

THE LEAN LIFESTYLE WORKOUT

We all know that working out makes us feel and look better. But we don't always know the most effective types of work out regimens. In the past, the recommendation for exercise was vague. Most people are very familiar with the past recommendation was thirty minutes of physical activity (moderate intensity) for the majority days of the week. However, research throughout the years has drastically changed the way we approach and recommend work out routines.

Currently, the weekly recommendation for physical activity (for people aged 18 to 65) is two and a half hours of aerobic (moderate) physical activity in addition to muscle strengthening (such as resistance training or weight lifting) on two or more days. These types of activities will be defined and illustrated in this chapter for a clear illustration of the regimens that are effective in improving mood, energy levels, and overall health. Discover a whole new way to revitalize your routine.

Spin!

"Spinning" (known officially as indoor cycling) has become increasingly popular among health conscious individuals. Spinning combines cardio and strength training supported by evidence. There is typically motivating music to move you toward your satisfying finish. While you sprint and climb your way through indoor cycling sessions at your local gym, you'll increase your energy and endurance. Additionally, you will likely jump-start your metabolism and burn plenty of calories as a result of the energy that is required by "spinning." Indoor cycling helps in burning excess fats resulting in weight loss and is an ideal form of exercise.

The Spin Workout (30 min)

1. *Warm up on the bike (4 min)*

2. *Lean forward (after adding resistance) for twenty seconds and lean back for twenty seconds. Alternate for five minutes total. (5 min)*

3. *Pick up the speed. Try going faster at each zero second, fifteen second, thirty second marks then recover at forty-five second mark and repeat for a total of four and a half minutes (4:30 min)*

4. *Intervals thirty seconds on thirty seconds off (5 min)*

5. *Seated Hill Climb (3:30 mins)*

6. *Standing sprints (after adding resistance)fifteen seconds up, fifteen seconds seated (4:30 min)*

7. *Slow speed to moderate with seated fast speed (tempo) ride (4 min)*

8. *Up the resistance, stand for hill climb, moderate pace (3 min)*

9. *Stay standing after adding heavy resistance steep slow hill (4:30 min)*

10. *Lower the resistance and make sure to sprint to the end (2 min)*

11. *Cooling-down ride*

Music during spin session is essential! Find a good instructor at your local gym to take you to the next level.

Hit the Weights

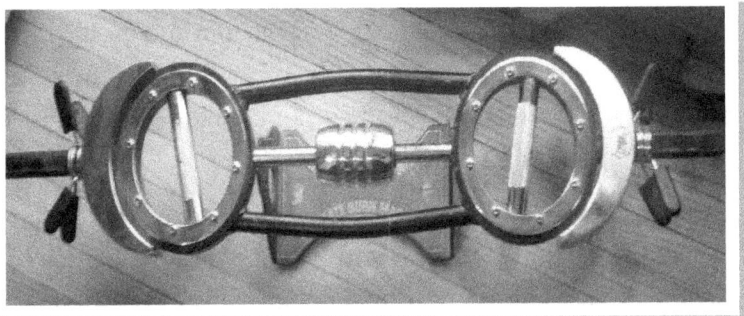

Given the current exercise recommendations and the research supporting the benefits of strength training, experts continue to stress the importance of engaging in some sort of resistance training in a weekly workout regimen. Even if you engage in aerobic activity on a regular basis, your muscles and bones will atrophy with age. Older people can greatly up their metabolism and prevent gaining weight by engaging in strength-training, such as weight lifting and other forms of fitness exercise.

The muscle contractions required during strength-training exercise consume additional metabolic energy and add to your total daily metabolic rate. After your strength training exercise, your metabolic rate will stay elevated for numerous hours as your muscles use additional metabolic energy to recover and grow. This can be helpful in contributing to a higher daily metabolic rate. As the percentage of muscle mass in your body increases (as the result of engaging in regular strength training) your daily resting metabolic rate will increase. If you have no idea how to begin this type of regimen, it is a great idea to hire a personal trainer for instruction and to prevent injury.

Two effective forms of strength training are circuit training and isometric training:

Isometric weight training involves activities such as holding a weight in one position for a given amount of time simply holding it up. One example of isometric weight training is simply holding a free weight straight in front of you for thirty to sixty seconds. Isometric training with weight has the ability to help with stamina improvement and make you stronger by holding the positions.

Circuit training: This type of training is ideal for the purpose of gaining strength as well as increasing endurance. Circuit training is very popular among fighters. This is due to the fact that it simulates what your body goes through in a wrestling or a boxing match.

The Circuit Training Workout (20 min):

1. *Pushups — maximum that you can complete in 1 minute*
2. *Squats — maximum that you can complete in 1 minute*
3. *Bicep curls with free weights — max in 1 min*
4. *Jog in place — max in 3 min*
5. *Bicep curls — max in 1 min*
6. *Lunges — 1 min per each leg (total 2 min)*
7. *Pushups — max in 1 min*
8. *Jog in place or jump rope — 3 min*
9. *Situps — 2 min*
10. *Lunges — 1 min per leg (total 2 min)*
11. *Bicep curls — max in 1 min*
12. *Situps — 2 min*
13. *Stretch*

*The important note about circuit training is to attempt to have little to no rest in between each set.

Splash!

No other workout boosts metabolism, burns calories, and firms every muscle in your body (without putting stress on your joints-it basically neutralizes gravity) better than swimming. Swimming is an excellent way to increase muscle tone as well as beneficial in strengthening muscles. This means that every swimming stroke becomes a resistance exercise, and as we are aware, resistance exercise is the optimal way to build muscle tone as well as strength. Whether you're a serious swimmer or simply looking for a non-impact workout, a swimming program designed specifically for you can be an effective way to improve your mind and body. The benefits of swimming on a regular basis include improvement in mood, an increase in energy levels and can even result in an added bonus of the highly desired "swimmer's physique".

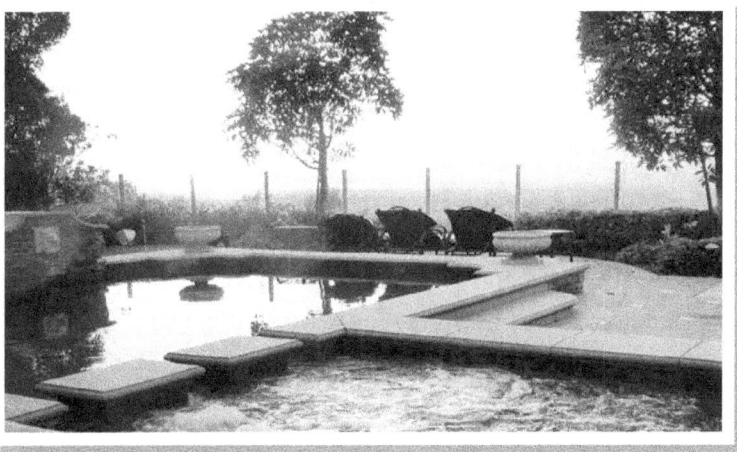

The Swimmer's Work Out:

A 5 by 100 is 100 yards, or four laps in a standard-sized pool, done five times.

Start your workout with a warm-up of six laps of freestyle and six laps of breaststroke. Keep your speed steady, you may increase it as you build endurance over time (in future workouts). Attempt to focus on your body position and breathing. Include basic sets such as 3 by 100 freestyle, 3 by 100 backstroke, 3 by 100 breaststroke or butterfly. Rest for 30 seconds between each set. This is a good standard swim workout, as you become stronger you can attempt to increase your speed!

Mind-body Training: Yoga and Tai Chi

Interestingly, effective workouts that can be done in the pool are yoga and Tai Chi. Many may not realize that yoga and Tai Chi can be practiced in the water. Whether you practice yoga in water or on dry land, you'll most likely enjoy health benefits with these "mindful" exercises. In private practice, I often recommend mindful exercises such as Tai Chi and yoga for stress and anxiety relief as well as relief from depressive symptoms. Tai Chi and yoga are known for health benefits (mental and physical), with very low risk to individuals even with medical problems. They are also known to increase flexibility and balance which are essentials for you workout regimen.

Both yoga and Tai Chi are mind-body training are supported by evidence-based extensive research and focus on engaging mentally, breath work, and the quality of movement. Movement has the potential to be positively life-altering. When approached in a conscious way, it can decrease anxiety and stress. Movement can also enhance weight loss, improve mood, and increase relaxation. It is essential to find effective ways to fully harness the power of the connection (mind-body) to reach your absolute potential.

Certified Health & Transformational Coach, Tiarra McLelland, asserts that yoga helps the mind as well as the body and can provide many different benefits to the person practicing, depending on where they are in their own personal healing journey. She adds that there are many different types of yoga to suit any fitness level and any age group and it is simply a matter of discovering the certain style that works best with you. Yoga expert Alexandra Indaco adds "Yoga is really about leaving all excuses behind and getting yourself to work, polishing the diamond, and not being afraid any longer of your own shining light."

According to Tiarra McLelland, yoga has a wide array of health benefits. The Benefits from yoga are: relief from anxiety as well as depression, cleansing of the body, calming of the mind, more flexibility, boost of the immune system, and reduction of the symptoms of certain chronic illnesses. Tiarra has known people who have healed long term chronic conditions from a regular yoga practice to people who simply were happy that they were finally able to fall asleep and stay asleep throughout the night. Additionally, a regular practice can get your body moving and burning calories, but also from a spiritual and emotional aspect may encourage one to address any eating and weight issues on a deeper level.

As a Certified Health & Transformational Coach, Tiarra's advice for someone starting out with mindfulness-based exercise is to take action and trust your intuition to guiding you to the right place to practice. She adds that there are many places with many forms but you must really pay attention to which one grabs your attention. If the first place doesn't fit then try another. She feels strongly that there is a certain type of yoga for everyone. It's really a matter of finding a place which resonates with you. Also, once you are in a class, make sure to not compare yourself to the person next to you. We are all on our own unique journeys, and it's about honoring yourself and body wherever it is at that moment. *Do your best and leave feeling happy.*

In addition to yoga, another notable form of exercise that can be done "mindfully" is walking. Walking is the frequent mode of physical fitness activity recommended professional medical settings. Moreover, according to the research, walking may be more adhered to than other exercises. Research has shown in studies that have examined minimally-active women that remaining with a program was higher with a walking group in comparison with a yoga group. Therefore, mixing up your routine with walking, yoga, and even more exercises could be a great way to stay engaged with your workouts.

Although walking is the most frequent mode of physical fitness activity recommended by health care professionals, mixed exercise (aerobic and resistance) is more effective than aerobic exercise alone in reducing patient-perceived symptoms of depression. In health care settings, advice from a medical professional can result in short-term (less than 12 weeks) increases in physical activity. However, referrals to exercise specialists can lead to long-term (up to eight months) change in both health care and community settings. Utilizing pedometers to measure number of steps.

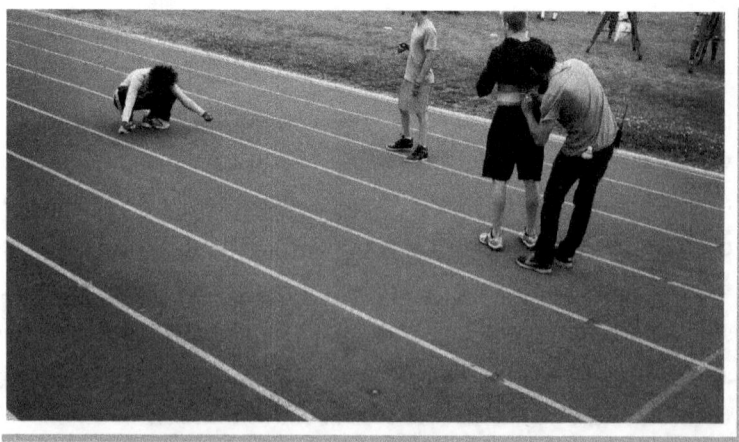

It is important for individuals to track their mood to acknowledge changes in energy levels. Mood logs are known to be beneficial in tracking a person's mood before and after exercise. A prominent researcher (Dr. Robert Thayer) had clients walk daily for thirty days while wearing pedometers. At the end of each day, every client was assessed for the number of steps taken and the changes in mood documented in the mood logs. According to the researcher, at the end of thirty days, clients reported feeling more energized, improved mood, and higher self-esteem.

The motivation to exercise can be sparked by short bouts of exercise. According to researchers, walking a mere 20 to 50 feet can energize individuals and have a positive impact on their mood. These short bouts of exercise can actually override a person's impulse to remain inactive. People should begin with a small amount of exercise at first and gradually increase the routine over time. Even a small amount of exercise has the potential to activate clients and improve mood. Short bouts of exercise can override your impulse to remain inactive. Therefore, it is highly recommended that you begin your physical activity regimens with brief time periods whether you are getting back into exercising or starting out for the first time.

Mind-Body Training: Pilates

Pilates is mind-body connection form of exercise. Pilates is a type of workout that is highly beneficial mentally and physically and taught on an international level. This exercise workout has six core principles: for centering, for concentration, for precision, for control, for flow, as well as for breath. These core purposes of Pilates exemplify the relationship between the mind and body that often results in an outcome of enhanced self-esteem and overall life satisfaction. Pilates can be done in the comfort of your home with videos or at your local Pilates studio.

A Favorite Pilates Move for Toning:

"TheBridge"

1. First, lie down with your knees bent and your feet planted on the floor

2. Then, push your hips as high as possible and hold them there

3. Next, take a deep breath in, and as you exhale, squeeze your glutes and pull your navel in toward your spine to make your torso as flat as possible while staying high as you can

4. You can maintain this tabletop torso by continuing to squeeze your glutes and abs

*You'll feel a good burn in the back of your legs (hamstrings) and in your glutes

Building your Personalized Workout Regimen

Systematic studies have been done on the most effective way of dealing with low energy, fatigue, and lack of motivation that negatively affects a person's ability to participate and benefit from physical activity. Strategies to improve physical activity participation levels that have been very helpful in healthy subjects can be utilized for people struggling with depression. It is essential for clients with factors of risk for cardiovascular disease to obtain a medical clearance before participating in a physical activity regimen. Additionally, the (PAR-Q) which is the physical fitness activity readiness questionnaire should be used in pre-participation screening for physical fitness (moderate) activity programs.

Physical activity can create a sense of accomplishment in clients that contributes to improved self-esteem. Cognitive override occurs when you gain knowledge about how to facilitate control over your mood by engaging in exercise, which prompts you to continue engaging in exercise to regulate your mood. Engaging in regular exercise results in increased energy, reduced tension and irritability, enhanced mood, and improved self-esteem.

Pay attention to your body and mood to gauge the most appropriate and effective types of exercise for yourself. Individuals with medical issues may need to slowly ease into exercise programs. The exercise regimens should be individualized and that physical difficulties should be considered. It is recommended that you consult a doctor who knows your health history before beginning any fitness regimen. Gentle activities for individuals with joint pain or previous injuries are also recommended.

For most people, six days a week of exercise with one day off is recommended. A workout regimen full of fun and variety (whether it involves walking, Pilates, yoga, Tai Chi, weight lifting, stationary biking, swimming, a combination thereof, or another challenging activity) is ideal. Variety is often essential, thus, you may opt to build several of the workouts in this chapter into your routine. The weekly routine should include aerobic activity, strength training, as well as balance and flexibility. The overall strategy should include activities you enjoy that will be sustainable long-term. Which activities will you choose for your regimen?

As a FREE bonus for this book you have exclusive access to your own Fitness Plan (7-day Workout) at the end of the book.

CUSTOMIZED WORKOUT PLAN

Day one:

Day two:

Day three:

Day four:

Day five:

Day six:

Day seven:

*At minimum, a single day out of the week should be a rest/ relaxation day!

PART III

Adopting the Fitness Motivation Mentality

Chapter Seven

ESTABLISHING FITNESS MOTIVATION-PROMOTING HABITS

The exercise-mental health connection is impossible to ignore due to the mounting evidence of the boost exercise brings to people. The new research regarding exercise and mood encourages therapists to do a better job of helping clients integrate exercise into their daily lives and help them to modify their activity regimens.

As a therapist, and as someone well aware of the mental health benefits of physical activity, I light up when my clients tell me about their weekend hikes, daily walks, or new sports for which they have recently taken back up. Just knowing that they're moving their muscles makes me excited because I know that they are utilizing one of the most effective tools for reducing depressive and anxiety symptoms. Even if you aren't currently depressed, you likely experience stress from time to time. In these situations you are likely to experience fight-or-flight sensations (i.e. heavy perspiration and increased heart rate) that may be unpleasant. Exercise can work as a sort of exposure therapy helping you to associate the fight-or-flight symptoms (i.e. heavy perspiration and increased heart rate) with safety instead of danger. This association can help immensely in stressful times.

Now that you are well equipped with the information regarding not only the physical benefits of exercise as well as the exercise-mental health connection, you will be given exciting and practical fitness motivating habits.

What is the Underlying Motivator for People to Exercise?

Consider the following factors that motivate people to not only begin but also stay with their workout program. Be sure to keep track of the ones for which you most likely relate.

► **Attractiveness:** Many long for improvements in appearance and a desire to become lean (results that can be obtained from weights lifting which firms the body, decreases the fat, and can increase the metabolism helping in weight control). Not only can you gain a leaner appearance, but your skin may also benefit from a consistent workout regimen. According to skin care professionals, you can rid your face of dirt and oil through regular workouts. You can take great satisfaction in these gains. May you look and feel fantastic!

► **Weight Loss:** Most people want a hot and healthy body. We want to fit into smaller sizes and feel comfortable in our clothes We live in a body-conscious society that makes us want to look great in a fitted clothes and swimsuits. The desire to be attractive often equates to people wanting to lose weight. One of the biggest industries is weight loss. It's big business and it's getting bigger all the time.

The worth of the weight loss industry has recently been estimated in the tens of billions of dollars.

Many lose control when they eat, they binge eat, and consume too many calories. It's essential that you're eating behaviors are healthy just like your exercise behaviors. Changing your lifestyle and your body will show you that you can control your life and all that it involves. We all know what it's like to lose control in some area of our lives. The key to weight loss is taking back control. When everything feels out of control in our lives, adhering to a healthy lifestyle is an important way to feel centered and focused, relaxed, and self-assured. Losing pounds of fat and fitting into a smaller size helps to instill confidence while aiding in wellness (as long as you are not restricting your calories with unrealistic diets). There are three principles that must be adhered to for successful weight loss:

1. Maintain a regular fitness routine

2. Watch your caloric intake-Do not diet or restrict too many calories and stay within your recommended range

3. Mix it up- keep your routines varied and fun

▶ **Enhanced Self-Confidence:** Confident people radiate a particular physical appeal and as well as charisma. I have noticed often times in my clinical practice that those who began a regular exercise program increased their self-concept, their physical abilities and wellness, and their health compared with people who stayed home. The most important factor was that their self-esteem increased right away even before they saw a marked physical change. It is merely a short jump to enjoying a healthier self-concept. Our self-esteem is very much tied to our energy levels. It is also tied to our feelings of ability and our perceived attractiveness. There is nothing much more appealing than the assurance about self that comes from feeling good in your body.

▶ **De-Stress:** Those who are feeling down or are experiencing stress often play with their mood by exercising. We know that exercise boosts feel-good neurochemicals in the brain. Your HPA axis serves the purpose of regulating your body's stress response through the process of releasing several types of (stress) hormones. Moreover, an HPA axis is known to not function normally in individuals with major depression. As a result of physical (exercise) and psychological stress, stress hormones are released by the HPA axis. Negative moods are associated with high levels of stress. Although overtraining increases stress hormone release, moderate training decreases the stress hormone release. Choose a workout routine that helps you de-stress and that fits your personality best.

▶ **Pleasure:** People often enjoy the actual act of working out whether it involves running, dancing, sports, or lifting weights. Many people claim they don't enjoy exercising. According to the research, before a workout, people underestimate the pleasure they'll derive from it. Before starting an hour-long workout session at a gym, predict on a scale of one to ten how much you expect to enjoy yourself. Then rate your satisfaction level at the end of the workout on a scale of one to ten (10 being the highest level of satisfaction). According to the research, you will likely wind up having significantly more fun than you originally expected, regardless of exercise intensity, and whether it's with cardio, yoga, Pilates, or another stimulating activity. People who workout regularly report greater expectations of satisfaction. The better you feel, the stronger your intentions will become to exercise on a regular basis. This is why I stress the importance of mixing your routines up and finding workouts you *truly* enjoy!

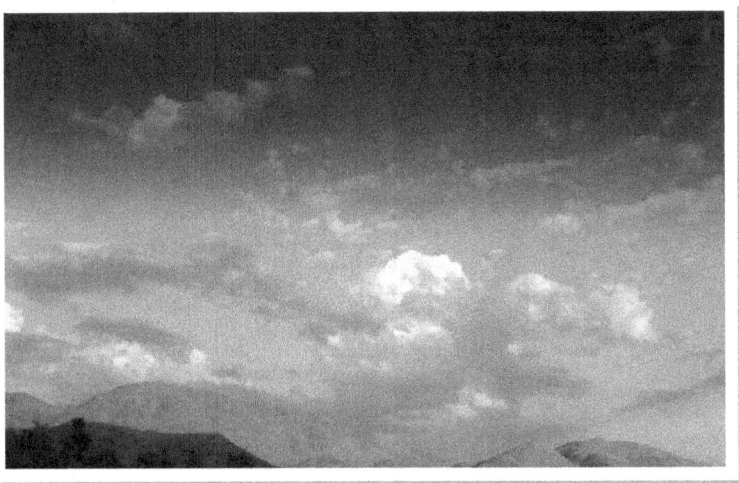

▶ **Fitness and Health Improvements:** Strength training increases muscle production as well as bone density. Exercise (overall) makes you feel stronger and increases your energy levels. It also helps promote sleep at night. Exercise can actually help prevent an onset of certain diseases as well as ease their symptoms.

▶ **Better Relationships:** researchers and practitioners of exercise assert that fitness activity engagement may enhance sexual experience as well as sexual performance. It has been shown by research that more time spent working-out is associated with a higher frequency (reported) of desired sexual activity. Physical endurance and muscle tone all improve sexual functioning.

▶ **Thrills:** Thrills from physical activity can be discovered at any age. Research shows that individuals who begin weight lifting or other forms of weight resistance later years of life find that they are able to attempt new and exciting activities like windsurfing or my favorite… kayaking.

▶ **Social Opportunities:** Working-out with your friends and/or family gives you an opportunity to visit and catch up while you workout. In these busy times, it's often essential that we are a able to get in more than one activity at a time. Here's a peek into ways to get you (and keep you) working-out:

▶ **Get Visually Inspired:** When I first started working out at the age of twenty-two, I remember finding a photo of a fitness model named Carmen and imagining myself with a similar physique. She had been interviewed by an online fitness magazine. I followed her diet plan exactly and stayed active six days a week (as she did) and happily reached my ideal body type. I've always believed in obtaining visuals for inspiration. A favorite workout magazine of mine is *Fitness Rx*, however, you may find other magazines that suit your ideal body types and there are plenty of online magazines and blogs today. If you surround yourself with visual cues, you have a great chance of meeting that goal. Frequently seeing bodies that you admire can motivate you daily to eat the healthiest and train the hardest. You will constantly see the people in the place where you want to be which will help get you there!

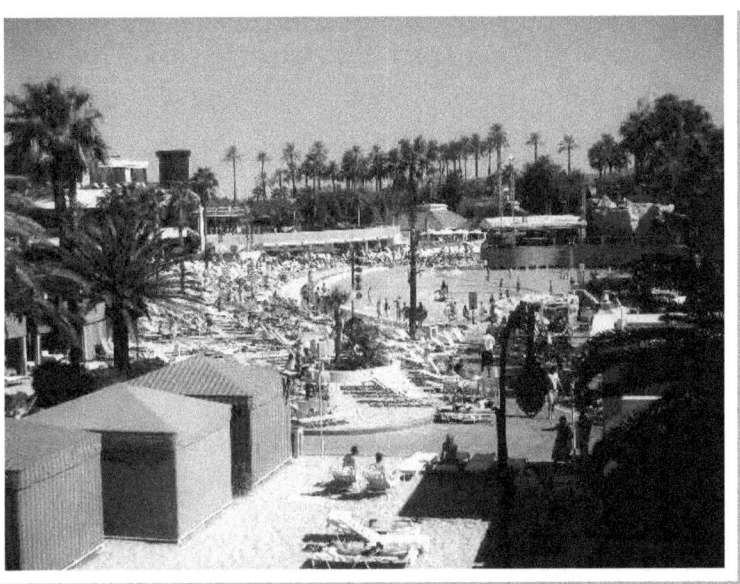

▶ **Schedule a Video Viewing:** Pre-workout, open a web browser, click YouTube, then search motivational videos. You will likely feel your eyes widening and your focus increasing. Videos help in many ways-- the background music can put you in happy and/or energetic moods, the motivational words while the video plays can inspire, and actually watching the fitness experts perform routines can make you want to repeat the moves in the gym. Even when I'm not in the mood to workout, all I have to do is open up my playlist and watch two to three of these videos and, minutes later, I'll be in the gym with weights in my hands. You can make your own playlist in YouTube with both music videos with your favorite artists that get you amped up and fitness videos that show you new routines. The option to change up your playlist can keep you stimulated and motivated to workout **all the time**! It makes no difference what activity you're engaged in, you can search that activity in YouTube which can make you work harder toward your goal.

▶ **Check Yourself Out:** I hesitated to write my personal experience in this realm, however, I'll sacrifice the uncomfortable feeling with hopes that someone reading this will use this as the motivational technique that I know is effective! Here it goes... when I started working out, I would come home from my session, take off my shirt (still with sports bra on) and stare. Why did I do this? Ego? Not exactly. It's like an unfinished art project... you visualize the next move/addition you would like to make. Are your arms more defined? Do you hold some extra fat you want to shed? It's self-defeating to be ashamed of taking a peek at your physique. Go ahead and stand in front of a mirror (I guarantee the person you look up to with the ideal energy level and physique does it). Whether you aren't yet proud of your physique, or you are satisfied, but want to improve, or you're loving your look -- checking your "project" out frequently can boost motivation. Tear that shirt off, check yourself out, and set goals of how you want to look!

▶ **Get the Right Workout Clothes:** Some believe exercise clothes do not make a difference in the potential for being successful and consistent in a workout routine. Many reasons are behind the importance of taking some time to pick out your workout attire. For instance, clothes can promote chafing that may deter a return visit to a next potential visit to a gym. If your outfit is even a bit uncomfortable, it is much easier to throw in the towel and cut your workout short.

Look the part!

It is easier to feel good about working-out (for most people) when you look good. You will get an extra boost in the gym if you feel comfortable and good about yourself. Be sure to choose clothing with your preferred fit, color, style, and material. Envision yourself as a professional runner, cyclist, or other sports figure when you select your work-out attire. The more you look like an athlete the more you will feel like an athlete, the more you feel like an athlete… the more you will behave like an athlete!

Need more potential gains to lace up your sneakers and maintain your routine? Here are a few more ways to ignite your fitness motivation:

▶ **Celebrate:** Making any lifestyle change can be challenging, to say the least. An excellent method of motivating yourself to keep with your workout routine is to adequately celebrate your achievements. Celebration is as important as visualizing success as well as setting goals. When you accomplish an important goal, ensure that you reward yourself adequately and well! Here are some great ways to celebrate your accomplishments:

1. **Throw a party for yourself (VIP style)**

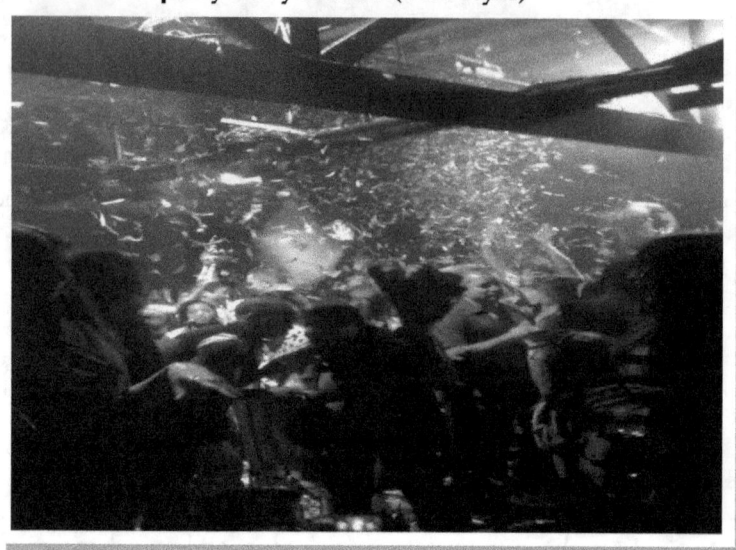

2. **Make plans with close friends to watch a movie or go hiking on a trail or near the beach**

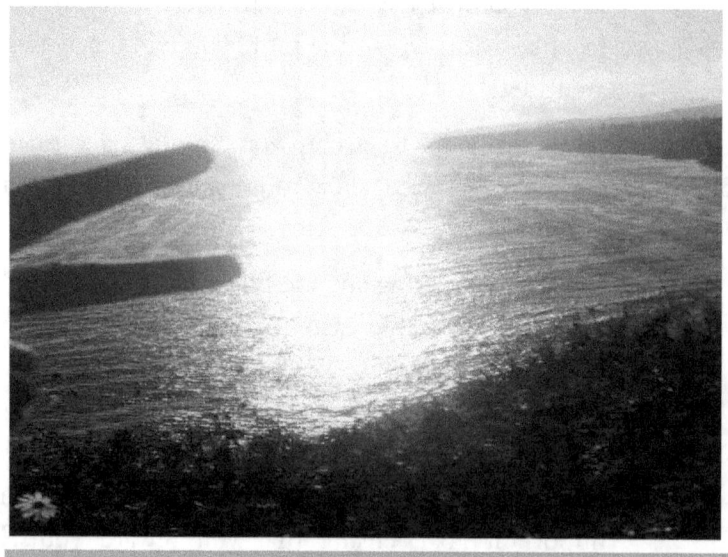

3. Go on a weekend getaway (plan this getaway when you begin setting your goals for motivation)

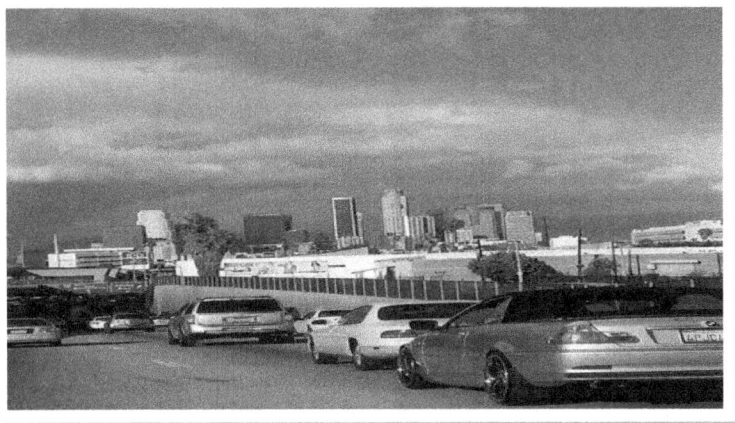

4. Obtain tickets to your favorite sports event, concert, or musical production

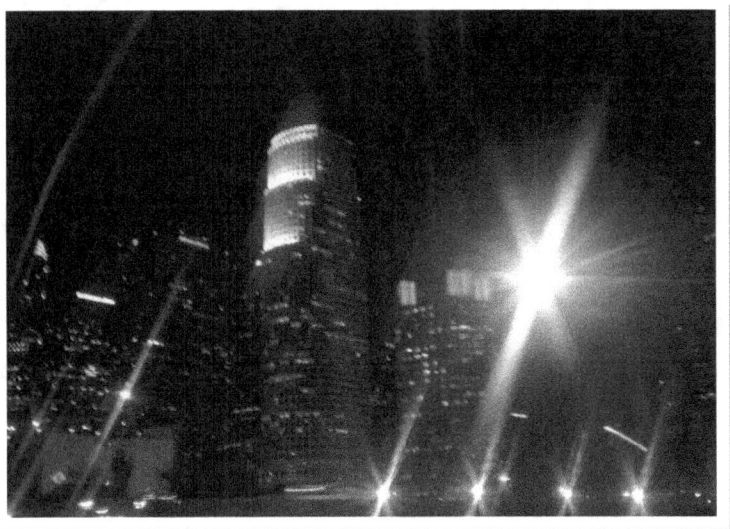

5. **Drive (or bike if you're close) to the beach**

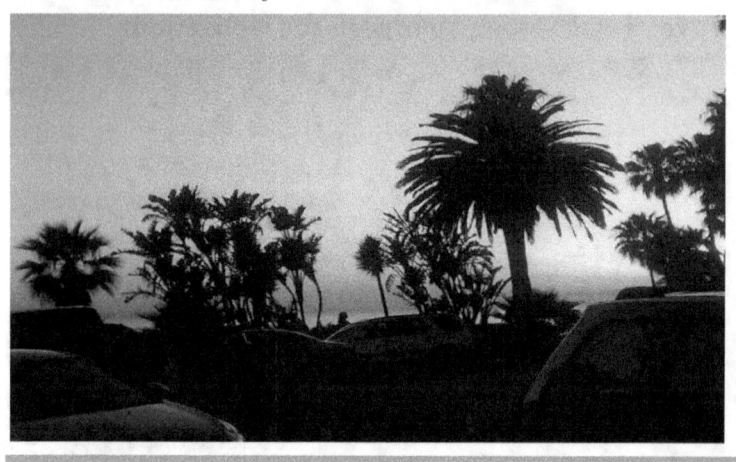

6. **Pamper yourself with a spa day (massage, manicure, pedicure, sauna, steam room)**

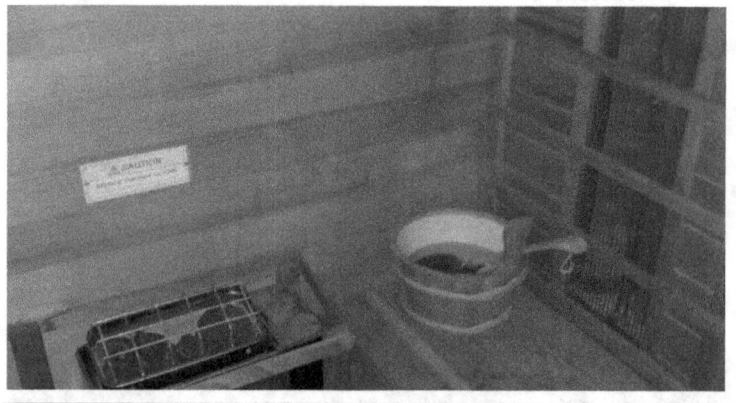

7. **Have professional photos taken**

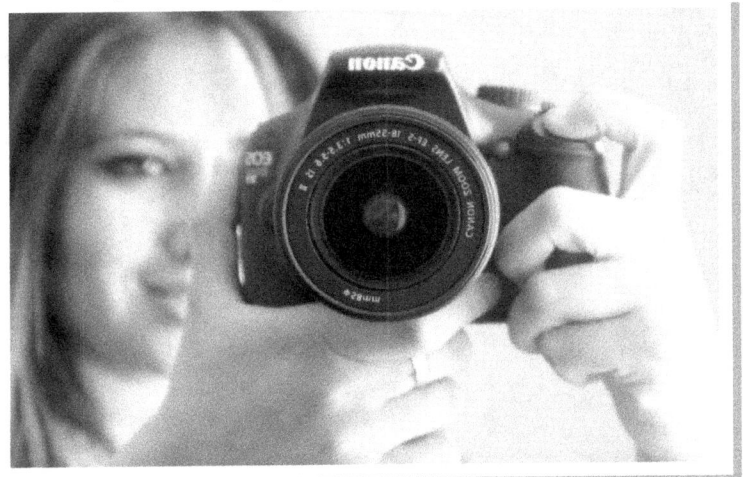

8. **Enroll in a class you've always wanted to go to (i.e. Zumba, Salsa dance, Spin etc.)**

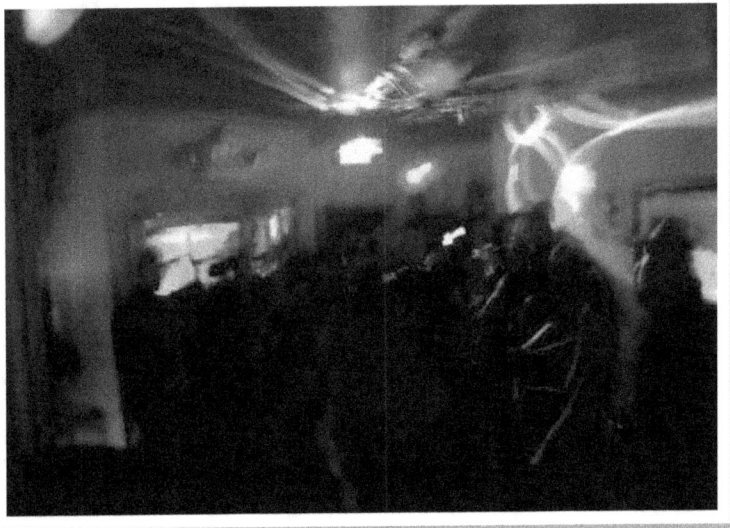

9. Go on a date to somewhere you've never been before

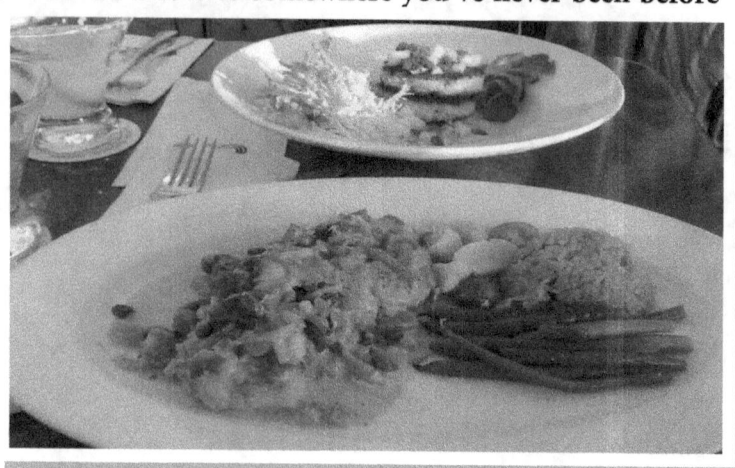

10. Take a day trip

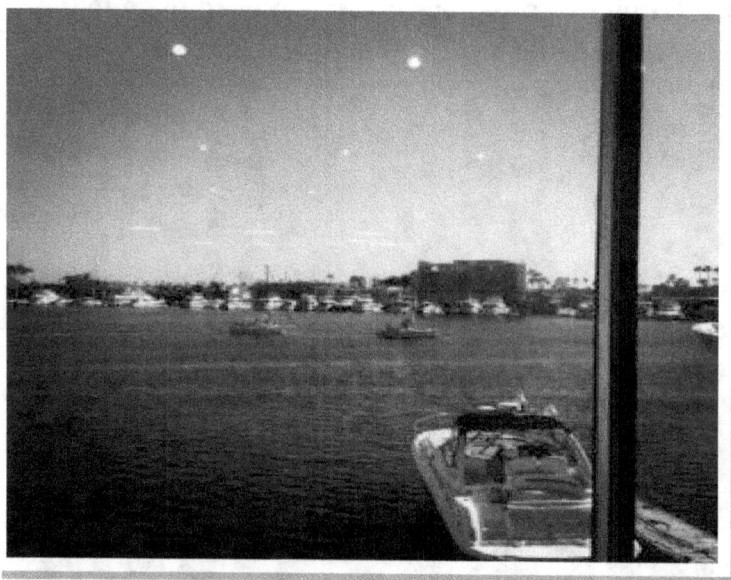

Enjoy your well-deserved celebration!

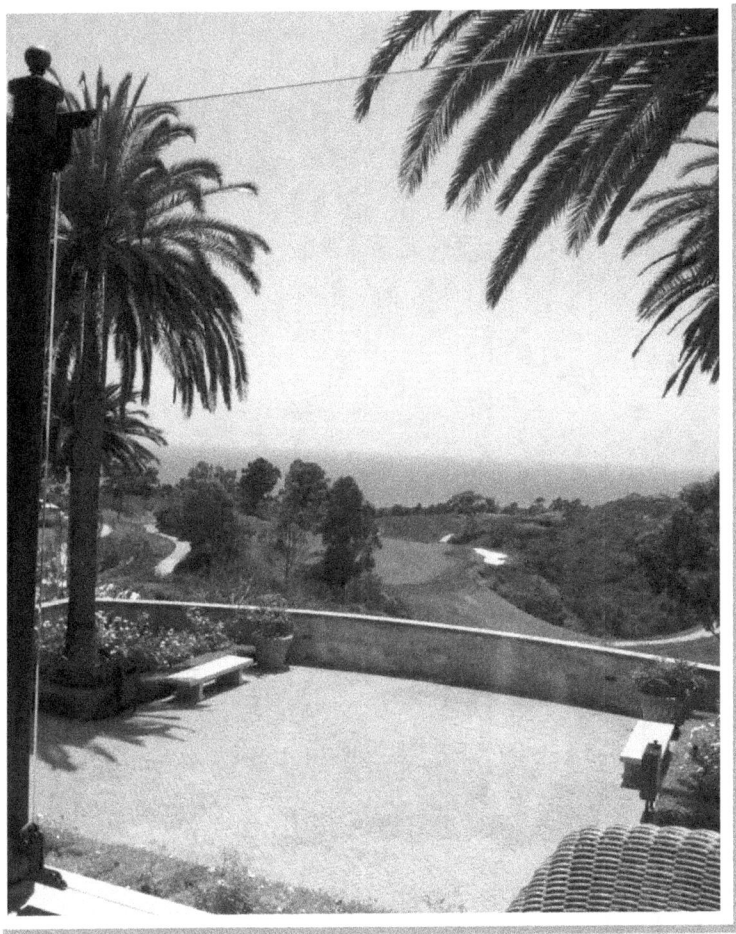

Chapter Eight

LEARNING TO THINK YOUR WAY TO A BETTER BODY

The Evidence-Based Intervention that Can Get You to Move

Cognitive Behavioral Therapy (CBT) is an action-oriented therapeutic intervention widely used by therapists and proven to be highly effective in modifying thoughts and behaviors. After reading about CBT and how it can help affect behavioral change (i.e. get you to exercise more often) you may decide to seek out a mental health professional for CBT therapy or you may simply utilize the tools provided at the end of this chapter. CBT is often used with clients for anxiety and depressive disorders, however, we will be discussing ways in which CBT can help to increase adaptive behaviors such as exercise (which in turn can increase mood and help to de-stress).

Self-talk. We can utilize positive self-talk to correct habits, improve self-confidence, and maintain fitness activity participation. Positive self-statements affect self-esteem in either a positive or negative way. Negative self-talk makes apparent exaggerated self-doubt such as the belief that they have no chance at succeeding in an exercise program. You alone control self-talk (how you choose to talk to yourself on a daily basis). Establishing and putting into practice positive self-talk can be a significant life-changing experience. We must become aware of our negative self-talk as well as alternative positive self-talk.

Often, people who are depressed report being unaware of their negative self-talk during physical activity. According to the research, in cases in which clients cannot accurately recall self-talk, a CBT activity such as daily reflections written down in your self-talk log can increase adaptive self-talk. This type of self-talk journaling can have in it the environment/location in which it happened and the emotional and/or performance consequences. Journaling typically helps for the most optimal highlighting of the triggers and consequences of self-talk as well as the greatest awareness of self-talk. Additionally, it may be beneficial for you to occasionally tape record yourself during exercise to document your self-talk.

Changing self-talk. When the previously noted interventions are utilized and you become aware of your self-talk, you may use interventions to alter your self-talk. The following techniques can be used to modify self-talk: re-phrasing negative thoughts to positive, thought stoppage, and lastly reframing. When you have finally committed to the change, some people will still struggle with reframing negative self-talk. When you find yourself in this situation, it is necessary for a mental health professional to look out for factors contributing to your difficulty in changing negative self-talk, i.e. low self-esteem or negative self-concept.

After you have identified self-statements that need elimination, the self-talk can be minimized with the technique of thought stoppage. Thought stoppage involves triggers that may be verbal (i.e., (a) **word "stop"**) or physical (i.e., (b) **clapping**).

The technique stops the undesired thoughts and may prevent negative self-talk with practice long-term. As a result, the negative self-talk can be stopped before it leads to negative feelings and behaviors such as discontinuing exercise.

In order to increase effectiveness you may need to (not only stop negative cognitions) but also follow them with a positive cognition. You may seem to have difficulty focusing for an enough length of time. You may keep falling back into previous ways of thinking even without trying and thus squash your most important intentions in just days, or even hours. Killing your good intentions results in a lack of manifestation. If you aren't content with the way your mind and body is now: intend change. Know that what you think about intently can result in attainment of results and we all wants results!

Thoughts control decisions which end up controlling results. When understood, you can begin to assume a great level of respect for your thoughts. You can decide to obtain control of your own thoughts. You may see that you are unwilling to simply accept what you don't want (like an out of shape body). It is important to develop an apparent and lasting respect for the power that intention has for your life.

As you are achieving your desires faster than ever before, you may feel inclined to engage in more and more thinking, feeling, acting, as well as meditating in a manner that is aligned with your goals. It is recommended that you spend about thirty or so minutes per day holding intentions with positive feelings and allowing them to circle around and marinade in your imagination.

Someone may assert, "I hate doing cardio," and this person might counter the assertion with, "I'm excited for my new adventure." Reframing can help create an accurate perspective on performance. Reframing, along with other techniques, can be effective in modifying self-talk but it is important to address the beliefs underlying the negative statements. Self-talk can be modified most effectively when a combination of stopping thoughts, countering, and reframing negative thoughts to positive thoughts is employed.

Research shows that cognitive-behavioral skills may have the best long-term effects in increasing physical activity participation for individuals. Cognitive-behavioral approaches are goal-oriented, present-centered, and time-limited. CBT is meant to be short-term and helps people gain the tools to motivate themselves to implement and maintain positive behavioral change such as engaging in regular exercise. In general, cognitive-behavioral strategies can be effective in motivating people to exercise and the approach should be encouraged in not only clinical settings but also made available to the general public. The CBT exercises provided for you here will be essential in helping you on your path to fitness drive initiation and maintenance.

COGNITIVE BEHAVIORAL THERAPY

The main concept of CBT is that *thoughts influence feelings* and *feelings influence behavior*. According to CBT, events don't cause feelings- our interpretation of events cause feelings. If we learn to replace automatic thoughts that are negative (such as, "I can never be fit") with more positive thoughts (such as, "I can everything I set my mind to") our emotional reactions will be more tempered and our behavior will be aligned with the positive more productive thought, therefore resulting in adaptive behaviors, such as engaging in physical activity.

COGNITIVE BEHAVIORAL THERAPY

Activity 1
Self-Talk Log

We need to get a sense of the negative thoughts that are no longer helping you in your journey to become motivated in your life. The self-talk log should include negative thoughts that you have about anything related to your ability, self-worth, performance, etc. The self-log should include the emotional and/or performance consequences. Additionally, it may be beneficial for you to occasionally tape record during exercise to document their verbalizations (See self-talk log on next page).

SELF-TALK LOG

Negative Thought   **Location/Trigger**

_____   _____

_____   _____

_____   _____

_____   _____

_____   _____

_____   _____

_____   _____

_____   _____

_____   _____

_____   _____

_____   _____

_____   _____

_____   _____

COGNITIVE BEHAVIORAL THERAPY

Activity 2
Reframing Self-Talk

Now that we have identified the negative self-talk that is preventing you from thriving, we can move onto positively reframing your thoughts. Reframing is a CBT technique of replacing negative self-talk to positive self-talk by writing down negative thoughts that we hold about ourselves and situations. When reframing, we re-write our self-talk in a more rational way.

Identify 8 of your most common destructive negative thoughts from the previous exercise and reframe with positive thoughts.

Negative Thought   Positive Thought
                                   to Replace

_____   _____

_____   _____

_____   _____

_____   _____

_____   _____

_____   _____

_____   _____

COGNITIVE BEHAVIORAL THERAPY

Activity 3
New Positive Affirmations

For ideal results repeat the affirmations before you head out to your workout so that they are fresh in your mind. You may even post them on your social media (many inspirational quotes can be found in apps on your phone or on the internet), save one as your screen saver, or print it out and put it up on your wall! Using these affirmations will get your mind in the right place, boost your motivation, and ensure that you push yourself. These affirmations will help you along your way to your ultimate fitness goals!

Being fit and vital is one of my top priorities in my life.

I always find the time to exercise.

Daily exercise makes me feel more energetic throughout my day.

Daily exercise makes me attractive.

Every workout gets me closer to my perfect body.

Every day I become more agile.

Every day I obtain maximum results by upping the intensity of my work- outs.

Every day I look leaner.

Every day I maximize my potential.

Every day my body becomes stronger and leaner.

Every day my body becomes younger.

Every day my muscles become more defined.

Every day my muscles grow stronger.

Exercise does as much for my mood as it does for my body.

Exercise greatly improves the way I feel about myself.

Exercise is the best stress relief.

Exercise is a powerful anti-depressant.

When I feel stressed or down I take a walk or head to the gym.

Exercise makes my body feel powerful.

Exercise makes me feel centered.

Exercise revitalizes my body and sharpens my mind.

Exercise tones up my body.

Exercising daily gives me increased energy.

Exercising is fun and enjoyable.

Exercising is rejuvenating; it brings me abundant energy.

Chapter Nine

Maintaining Mind and Body Enhancing Attitudes and Beliefs

Physical activity has been proven to help improve mood and energy levels. Despite the fact that regular physical activity has been shown so effective, only 25 percent of Americans participate in physical activity at the recommended level (by the CDC, the AHA, the ACSM, and the US Surgeon General) according to behavioral risk factor surveys. As a result, a large percentage of American adults don't actively participate in regular fitness regimens and thus do not benefit from the positive mental and physical health benefits of fitness.

Although exercise can be greatly beneficial to the mental health of clients, many depressed clients do not engage in enough physical activity and thus are not able to benefit from the mood-elevating effects caused by regular exercise. Many people often struggle to maintain the motivation necessary to participate in regular physical activity.

Scientists explain physical activity as being immensely beneficial to the mind and body. Every cell in the physical human body benefits from physical fitness activity. The rewards of fitness extend way beyond losing weight or adding muscle composition. Many changes visibly improve the body and mind in ways scientists are just beginning to figure out. Anyone who takes the initiative of forming a habit of going to the gym, unrolling a yoga mat, or hiking in the hills is aware of a secret revealed only to the active.

Final Motivational Tips

Change It Up

When you want your body to change, you have to change up your workouts. When you find yourself not making progress (known as plateauing) you have to make some changes. After about a month of staying consistent with your set routine, change it up-add a new class at your gym or simply choose one of the exercises outlined for you in this book and add it to your workout regimen. This will give your body new challenges and get you the results you want.

Get Into It with the Most Optimal Attitude

There is definite correlation between attitude and achievement. Be sure to go into working out with a trainer, or going to the gym or participating in a weight loss program with the best possible attitude. Good attitude equals a good outcome. It is possible to sabotage ourselves with a bad attitude. Over the years, I've witnessed people complain, blame (trainers call this "Blame the Trainer"), justify, and procrastinate and then end up feeling defeated with the same state in which they started. On the other hand, I have witnessed many people with limited time and money create and keep incredible results because they got their head in the game and kept it there. *My advice is… go in with the best possible attitude and leave with the best possible results.*

Control Your Thoughts for the Ultimate Body

Getting in shape is an internal process and much more of it than it is an external one. When we get the internal situation right… the external change is just a positive by-product. The mind is your biggest obstacle and your biggest asset when it comes to physical fitness. If you think about being overweight and worry constantly about your appearance then you are working against your goals. According to CBT, our thoughts affect our feelings and our feelings then affect our behavior. Your negative thoughts have been the cause of the unhappy feelings about yourself and maladaptive behaviors (such as not living up to your fitness potential). Change your thoughts to feel better and align your behaviors with those positive thoughts about yourself for some serious results!

Make Time for You!

Every day, or at a minimum, six days a week, do something for yourself that gets you moving. Let the people close to you know that that time is yours and can't be rescheduled. I know many CEOs that will not schedule a meeting at 7 am, for example, because their workout is at 6:30 and they cannot be interrupted. This time for yourself needs to be nonnegotiable. You are not being selfish by taking this time out for yourself. After giving so much time to family, friends, and work, everyone needs to recharge. In fact, this time out for yourself will make you more efficient in every aspect of your life. When you begin to get accustomed to this habit of making time for you, you will see a difference in your body, energy levels, and your mood. *It's not a matter of how many hours in the day, it's a matter of priorities.*

Just Do It

The famous saying "Just Do It" really does work. You can't overthink working out. You really have to get out there and get into it. Trying to convince yourself to work out too much has been proven to have a negative impact your motivation. The research shows it's more effective, once you've removed your self-defeating thoughts, to just get out there and work-out. If you only exercise when you're in the mood you'll never be maintain or be consistent and you'll never create long-lasting change. If you just do not feel like working-out, do it anyway. You may not love the process but you *will* embrace the results.

Keep Track of Your Progress

Make yourself accountable by writing down your routines before your workout. Get a journal to keep track of your routines and your progress each day. If you prefer to log everything on your phone you can use the free app called *JEFIT Workout* where you can log your exercises in your calendar daily. If you know you're expected to lift weights to help define your shoulders and triceps you will be more likely to follow through if it's written down in your log. It is absolutely motivating to see your strengths and improvements "on paper." When you see how much progress you've made looking back at your log you'll be inspired to continue on the fitness path.

Visualize

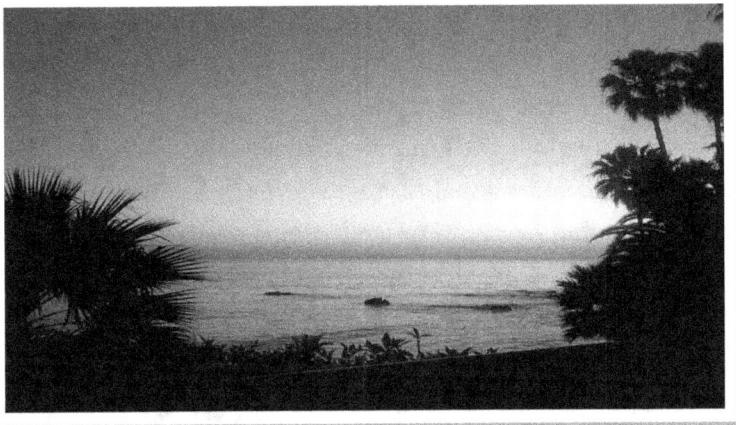

Put your mind in the place where it needs to go and your body will follow right alongside. Visualization techniques are effective and are based on the bio-psycho-social model in that thoughts create feelings and feelings have the capacity to affect the physiology of one's body as well as one's behaviors. For example, by engaging in such practices as placing a photo of yourself on the head of a representation of your ideal body and visualizing yourself actually having that body you will align your behavior with your ideal self.

You are no longer in a hoping or wishing mind frame when you see yourself already fit, happy and healthy. "Fake it 'til you make it" is a powerful tool that can propel you right in the direction of your fitness goals. You can assert to yourself that you have already attained your ideal body and energy levels before it manifests and this will have a positive impact on your ability to go all the way. You can assert present-tense phrases to yourself such as, "I am changing my body," or "I'm changing my life," or "I love my new body", and "I'm getting more fit every day."

You can walk taller with your chest out and shoulders back and start believing you are healthier now.

Training your mind with visualization can effectively catapult you to achieve your goals. When you begin to see yourself as a healthy, attractive, and desirable person, your behavior will align with this visualization and your work outs will increase. Start visualizing now. Imagine yourself working out and loving every minute. Imagine yourself going about your day in your ideal body. These visualization should be done daily. You will be incredibly satisfied by the results.

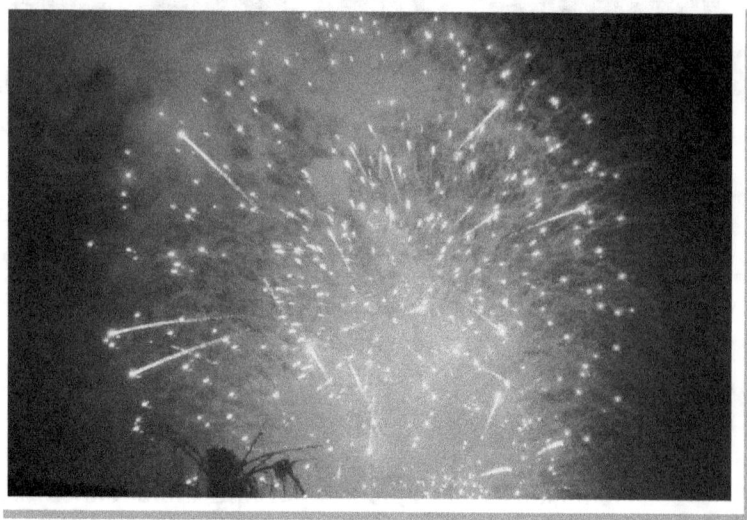

On Your Mark, Get Set...You're Almost There!

You are actively creating the body and mind, the energy and confidence that you've always desired. Your obstacles have been obliterated and you have all of the tools to get you up, inspired, and amped up for your regular workouts with the results. You no longer wish for a more attractive body and fulfilling life; you are now taking it and reaping the rewards for yourself. You have the tools for a higher quality of life. Your thoughts, feelings, and behaviors are creating this new life. Now that you have embraced this motivational outlook, new opportunities will be handed to you, obstacles will look like opportunities, and nothing will ever hold you back again. You have created a new mind and the body is following… aligning with your new thoughts, feelings, and behaviors. You have all of the power; you have everything you need, recognize your achievements and celebrate the new mind and body you have created.

…Go!

PART IV

Extras

BONUS 7-DAY WORKOUT

(Always consult your physician before beginning a new fitness regimen)

Day 1: Strength-Training and Cardio

*You will need free weights (either 5, 8, 10 or more lbs each depending on fitness level)

20 min on elliptical or treadmill (walk in neighborhood or hike if no equipment nearby)

3 sets of 15 deep squats (make sure not to allow knee to extend over toes)

3 sets of 12 pushups (can be modified version meaning on knees)

3 sets of 20 bicep curls (free weights in both hands i.e. 5 lb for beginner, 8-10 lbs each for moderate, and increased weight for advanced)

2 sets of 20 alternating lunges (which means 10 lunges on each side per set)

4 sets of 20 sit-ups

15 minutes on elliptical or treadmill (walk in neighborhood if no equipment nearby preferably hills)

Stretch and congratulate yourself!

Day 2: Cardio

Minimum 30 minutes

Take a class at a local gym for your workout on Day 2. These should be cardio classes such as spin (indoor cycling), Zumba, etc.

Day 3: Mind-Body Workout

Practice a minimum of 40 minutes of any of the following mind-body connection activities...

- yoga

- tai chi

- or pilates

Day 4: Strength-Training Only

3 sets of 20 shoulder presses

3 sets of 20 alternating lunges

3 sets of 20 chair dips (aka tricep dips) (can be done on weight bench, firm sofa or chair)

4 sets of 20 sit-ups

Hold plank position for 60 seconds

4 sets of 20 sit-ups

3 sets of 20 squats

Stretch

Day 5: Sport/Passion Workout

As discussed in *The Psychology Behind Fitness Motivation: A Revolutionary New Program to Lose Weight and Stay Fit for Life*, it is critical to find your favorite sport or other favorite activity that involves *cardio* and engage at least once a week.

Engage in at 40 minutes of the following types of cardio:

- Swimming

- Dancing (i.e. Zumba, Salsa, Merengue...)
- Basketball
- Tennis
- Racquet ball
- Kayaking

Day 6: Hiking

Take a 30 to 60 minute hike outdoors. You will be amazed how many calories you will burn while enjoying your surroundings!

Day 7: Rest and Rejuvenation

All of the biggest fitness industry experts will tell you that as much time as you dedicate to going hard on your body, you must balance it out with rest, repair, and rejuvenation.

Treat yourself to two of the following activities every Rest and Rejuvenation Day:

- Mindful Meditation
- Full body massage
- Reiki session
- Utilize a foam roller to release tension in your muscles
- Sit in a sauna
- Enjoy a steam room
- Soak in a hot bath
- Relax in a Jacuzzi at your gym or home

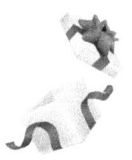 # COUPON CODES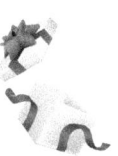

Here is the coupon for 40% off of the print version of the book:

Apply this coupon at checkout and receive 40% off the paperback version. Go here to the official createspace store to apply the discount:

http://www.

Coupon code: 64EEQA92

*Note, the discount code won't work if you buy the book from amazon, it will only work if you buy it from the createspace store as they are the distributor of the book.

References List

INTRODUCTION:

Chronister K. *How To Motivate Depressed Adult Clients To Engage In Physical Activity* [e-book]. US: ProQuest Information & Learning; 2012. Available from: PsycINFO, Ipswich, MA. Accessed October 27, 2013.

CHAPTER ONE:

Chronister K. *How To Motivate Depressed Adult Clients To Engage In Physical Activity* [e-book]. US: ProQuest Information & Learning; 2012. Available from: PsycINFO, Ipswich, MA. Accessed October 27, 2013.

CHAPTER TWO:

Chronister K. *How To Motivate Depressed Adult Clients To Engage In Physical Activity* [e-book]. US: ProQuest Information & Learning; 2012. Available from: PsycINFO, Ipswich, MA. Accessed October 27, 2013.

CHAPTER THREE:

Chronister K. *How To Motivate Depressed Adult Clients To Engage In Physical Activity* [e-book]. US: ProQuest Information & Learning; 2012. Available from: PsycINFO, Ipswich, MA. Accessed October 27, 2013.

CHAPTER FOUR:

Chronister K. *How To Motivate Depressed Adult Clients To Engage In Physical Activity* [e-book]. US: ProQuest Information & Learning; 2012. Available from: PsycINFO, Ipswich, MA. Accessed October 27, 2013.

CHAPTER FIVE:

Chronister K. *How To Motivate Depressed Adult Clients To Engage In Physical Activity* [e-book]. US: ProQuest Information & Learning; 2012. Available from: PsycINFO, Ipswich, MA. Accessed October 27, 2013.

CHAPTER SIX:

Chronister K. *How To Motivate Depressed Adult Clients To Engage In Physical Activity* [e-book]. US: ProQuest Information & Learning; 2012. Available from: PsycINFO, Ipswich, MA. Accessed October 27, 2013.

CHAPTER SEVEN:

Chronister K. *How To Motivate Depressed Adult Clients To Engage In Physical Activity* [e-book]. US: ProQuest Information & Learning; 2012. Available from: PsycINFO, Ipswich, MA. Accessed October 27, 2013.

CHAPTER EIGHT:

Chronister K. *How To Motivate Depressed Adult Clients To Engage In Physical Activity* [e-book]. US: ProQuest Information & Learning; 2012. Available from: PsycINFO, Ipswich, MA. Accessed October 27, 2013.

CHAPTER NINE:

Chronister K. *How To Motivate Depressed Adult Clients To Engage In Physical Activity* [e-book]. US: ProQuest Information & Learning; 2012. Available from: PsycINFO, Ipswich, MA. Accessed October 27, 2013.

---

*Photography for this book by Griselda Noriega; headshot by Hollywood Pro Photography

About the Author

Dr. Kim Chronister is an author, wellness expert, and health psychologist. Prior to becoming a health psychologist, Dr. Chronister worked as a certified personal trainer. During her undergraduate program she worked with clients as a certified personal trainer successfully improving the lives and well-being of many clients. While pursuing her doctoral degree, she provided individual, family, couples, and group therapy 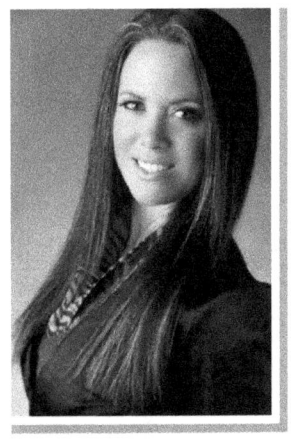 to clients suffering from substance abuse, eating disorders and other issues such as anxiety and depression in residential, community, and a psychiatric facility in southern California. She has gained experience utilizing cognitive behavioral therapy (CBT) with clients struggling with eating disorders (including binge eating disorder), interpersonal issues, substance abuse, anxiety, and depressive disorders. Additionally, she uses motivational interviewing (MI) to help clients gain motivation to engage in physical activity for the benefit of decreasing stress and improving mood. Dr. Chronister uses a strength-based approach to therapy and focuses on the strengths of individuals and couples rather than pathology.

As a wellness expert and health psychologist, Dr. Chronister has been asked to comment on subjects as overeating, exercise motivation, substance abuse, relationships, and fitness routines for popular magazines, books, and documentaries. She emphasizes in her clinical practice the importance of physical fitness activity on mood and overall well-being for individuals as well as couples. Dr. Kim Chronister currently provides therapy to clients in private practice of West Los Angeles, California.

DrKimChronister.com

www.ingramcontent.com/pod-product-compliance
Lightning Source LLC
Chambersburg PA
CBHW070921290526
45795CB00001B/376